SKIN CANCER

DR TOM SMITH has been writing full time since 1977, after spending six years in general practice and seven years in medical research. He writes regularly for medical journals and magazines, has a weekly column in the *Bradford Telegraph and Argus* and also writes for the *Lancashire Evening Telegraph* and the *Carrick and Galloway Gazettes*. He also broadcasts regularly for BBC Radio Scotland. His other books for Sheldon Press include *Heart Attacks: Prevent and Survive, Living with Alzheimer's Disease, Coping Successfully with Prostate Cancer, Overcoming Back Pain, Coping with Bowel Cancer* and *Coping with Heartburn and Reflux*.

Overcoming Common Problems Series

Selected titles

A full list of titles is available from Sheldon Press,
36 Causton Street, London SW1P 4ST, and on our website at
www.sheldonpress.co.uk

Overcoming Common Problems Series

Overcoming Common Problems Series

Overcoming Common Problems

Skin Cancer

Prevent and Survive

Dr Tom Smith

sheldon PRESS

First published in Great Britain in 2006

Sheldon Press
36 Causton Street
London SW1P 4ST

British Library Cataloguing-in-Publication Data
A catalogue record for this book is available from the British Library

ISBN-13: 978–0–85969–967–9
ISBN-10: 0–85969–967–6

1 3 5 7 9 10 8 6 4 2

Typeset by Deltatype Limited, Birkenhead, Merseyside
Printed in Great Britain by
Ashford Colour Press

Contents

Introduction

Skin cancer is the fastest-growing cancer in the UK and other countries with temperate climates, and this at a time when almost all other cancers are in decline. Part of the reason for the rise in skin cancer is that we are exposing ourselves far more to the sun than did previous generations. But, there is much more to skin cancer than the damage caused by the sun, or than health warnings about avoiding sunburn. This book is about all the common types of skin cancer, how they are recognized and diagnosed, how they are treated in the early and later stages, and the extent to which they can be prevented. It also offers high hopes for the future for cures of skin cancers, including the most malignant ones.

The common skin cancers form three main types, basal, squamous and melanoma, named from the cells in the skin that give rise to them. Below, I explain this classification. The different types of skin cancer have very different growth and spread patterns and, if not recognized and treated early enough, different outlooks.

For example, the basal cell cancer (BCC) arises mainly on the face in the triangle between eye, upper lip and ear, and does not spread distantly, although it can 'bore into' the face, leaving an unsightly ulcer. It is almost always completely cured. It is about three times more common than squamous cell cancer, which arises on skin that is repeatedly sun-exposed, such as the forehead and temple, the backs of the hands and the forearms, and does spread to distant organs, although slowly. Treated early it is usually curable, but it must not be left until it has spread elsewhere.

Melanoma arises anywhere, from the soles of the feet to the top of the head, and at sites that are unrelated to sun exposure. It spreads more widely and at an earlier stage than the other two cancers, and once it has been diagnosed it must be treated as an emergency. It is much more lethal than the other two types of cancer, and needs very specialized treatment. The new research into forms of treatment of melanoma takes up a substantial part of this book.

Skin cancer is scary because it is so obvious: it frightens us because we can see it. That makes it different from cancers of the internal organs, which may be growing slowly for some months before their eventual size or spread elsewhere make their presence felt. So although we fear skin cancer, most of the time we recognize it early enough to have it diagnosed and treated. Nowadays, people don't delay in seeking advice when they notice any small change in the skin – such as a new 'freckle' or a change in a 'mole' or a small 'pit' appearing in the face – and doctors like myself, who have been around for more years than they like to admit, see cases in a much earlier stage of development than they used to.

The recent publicity about skin cancers that has concentrated mainly on the link with exposure to the sun has made us much more aware than our parents were of subtle changes in our skin. Recognizing early skin cancer in its initial stages, even before it becomes truly cancerous, is a huge advantage, particularly for melanoma, as cure, and therefore survival, may depend on early and complete treatment.

This is an optimistic book: most people with skin cancer are seen early and treated comprehensively at a stage when it can still be eradicated. In the first chapter I use my memories of men and women in my years as a houseman and a family doctor to take you through the ways that skin cancers arise and develop. It gives a flavour of what a doctor has to do when faced with people whose skin problems may be cancers. It is more of a personal diary of cases than a medical text; I'm sure most GPs would agree that they have learnt much more about 'skins' once they started in practice, and were seeing patients every day, than they did at medical school. Annie's case (the first case history in Chapter 1) is a prime example of this self-education. Every doctor would have a similar tale to tell.

Examining skin is not a precise science: as with Annie, there are times when something looks malignant but is not. There are other occasions when something that looks benign is in fact potentially lethal. Often the only way to tell the difference is to remove the 'lesion' (our word for an area of skin that has become abnormal) and examine it under the microscope. That is a job, obviously, for the specialist dermatologist. So, after describing the construction of normal skin in Chapter 2, Chapter 3 explains how it changes with developing cancer, and has a short section on how specialists classify the changes.

Why skin cancers arise deserves a special chapter. We have been bombarded by warnings about exposure to the sun and how it may cause cancerous changes in the skin, and the evidence for them is laid out in Chapter 3. However, there is another side to the 'sun causes cancer' argument, and for the sake of balance I have included a defence of sunbathing in the same chapter. Chapter 4 describes the benign skin problems that many people mistake for cancer.

From Chapter 5 onwards, the book concentrates on the various types of skin cancer, first describing each cancer in turn, and then their treatments. Getting rid of a skin cancer isn't always a matter of just cutting it out. They can be burnt, frozen or injected away, as well as removed by a scalpel. They can also be made to disappear using chemical and immunological means, and these deserve a chapter to themselves.

Each type of skin cancer demands a different treatment approach, so the following chapters take them in turn, starting with basal cell cancers (commonly called rodent ulcers), continuing with squamous cell cancers, and concluding with melanoma. Much of what I describe as their current treatment is taken from my experience as a GP in the UK, but I also report on reviews published since 2003 in which skin cancer treatments in the UK and USA have been scrutinized and compared. They cover medical and surgical treatment of the initial cancers and also the comprehensive treatment of those that have spread (metastasized). Metastasis is not necessarily a death sentence, as it used to be, because of the recent development of immunotherapy that targets the cancer cells wherever they are.

I have devoted part of Chapter 3 to commenting on how the average person sees, or ignores, the threat of skin cancer, and to describe how health organizations in different countries have tried to promote public awareness about the risks of skin cancer. In December 2004, Martin Weinstock, of Brown University, Rhode Island, in the USA, described the most effective ways of educating the public about the different forms of skin cancer. He included advice on how to recognize them early, how to enjoy the sun without endangering your health, how to have a sensible approach to tanning, and how to estimate your own risk of skin cancers, including melanoma. The lifetime risk of a skin cancer is now an unbelievable 1 in 5, and that of melanoma is 1 in 74, so everyone needs to be aware of skin cancer and its symptoms.

No book on skin cancers can avoid controversy. There is current concern about sunscreens, with some researchers suggesting that putting on sunscreen means that people stay longer in the sun, and that this promotes, rather than protects against, skin cancer. This was discussed in detail in the professional journal of skin diseases, *Archives of Dermatology*, in June 2004, and I have based my practice and advice on sunscreens on that discussion.

A few rare skin cancers, such as mycosis fungoides and Bowen's disease, are treated in later chapters (Chapters 10 and 4 respectively). They need early recognition and treatment if the person is to survive, so the initial signs will be described in this chapter.

Future ways of preventing and treating skin cancers will also be reviewed. Research into skin cancers, and especially melanoma, has raised hopes for very specific treatments to eradicate not just the lesion in the skin, but also the secondary cancers ('metastases') that eventually threaten life. The book is therefore optimistic in tone, and I hope that readers with skin cancers will be reassured that they are living in an age when so much more can be done than was the case only a few years ago.

1

Changes in the skin

Annie

Annie was 24 when I met her. We were both new to the district – I was a young GP fresh from Birmingham, she was from Glasgow, and had married a shepherd the previous summer. The district? A Scottish farming community. The time? April. These details do matter, as the following paragraphs make clear.

Annie had a 'lesion' on her right wrist. It was about 1 centimetre across, was raised above the surrounding skin, was bright red and oozing a thick yellow pus from its centre. It was not in the least painful – possibly an ominous sign in any change in the skin that might be cancerous. Annie had noticed the 'lump' three or four days before, and it had developed rapidly, first as a red lump, then growing in size and in its degree of redness, and finally breaking down into an ulcer in its centre that was obviously infected. For my part, I felt the large ulcerating purulent painless lump could well be a rapidly advancing cancer, and I had to take urgent action.

I telephoned the hospital, about 50 miles away, and asked to speak to the dermatologist. We did not know each other – I had only been in the district a week – so I wasn't sure what to expect. I explained that I was worried about a young woman with a suspicious lesion on her wrist and described its appearance. I asked him if he could see her urgently. The conversation then took an unexpected turn:

Dermatologist: 'Where did you qualify, doctor?'
Me: 'Birmingham.'
Dermatologist: 'Not many sheep in Birmingham, then?'
Me (nonplussed): 'Er, no.'
Dermatologist: 'I think you'll find she has been feeding a lamb.'
Me: 'Well, she is a shepherd's wife, but what has that got to do with it?'
Dermatologist: 'Look up *orf* in your medical textbooks, then call me back.'

I hadn't heard of 'orf'. It is an infection of sheep caused by a virus of the same family as cowpox and smallpox. Lambs catch it from their mothers: it forms sores around their mouths. People catch it from close contact with the lamb – mostly from bottle-feeding an orphan lamb. The lambs recover quite quickly, but the person is left with a single large sore, exactly like Annie's, at the spot on the skin that has been in contact with the lamb's mouth. If you are old enough to remember a smallpox vaccination as a child, then you know exactly what it looks like. The textbooks of general medicine contain only a line or two about orf, and my dermatology textbook didn't mention it at all.

Annie hadn't known what it was because she was new to the district. If she had asked a neighbour, or even her husband (she had hidden it from him, not wanting to worry him), they would probably have been better informed about it than me.

Missing that diagnosis was a real embarrassment for me as a new doctor in the district, and I was determined not to repeat it. Tom Cochrane, the dermatologist, and I became good friends, and for many years I referred my skin patients to him, in the process learning much about spotting when a skin problem might be cancerous or be likely to become cancerous. Many of the patients I describe in the following paragraphs are from my time working with him.

James

James, a 63-year-old beef cattle farmer, had the ruddy complexion of a man who had spent most of his working life outdoors. He had several small lumps on his cheeks that were smooth and the same colour as the rest of his skin, caused him no pain or discomfort, and had been there for many years. They were probably the remains of his teenage acne, and contained the now-solid secretions of old inflamed glands. So he didn't take much notice when a new lump appeared on the side of his nose, in the fold between the fleshy part of his nostril and the side of his cheek. What was one more lump to add to the others, especially as it too wasn't bothering him in the least?

He only became concerned when the lump grew larger and, as it did so, changed in colour and shape. By the time it was the size of a small pea it had a dimple in the middle, making it the shape of a tiny doughnut, with the outer fleshy ring being red, and the inside edge having a pearly sheen that 'rolled over' into the centre. Tiny thread-like blood vessels were scattered over its surface and in the skin surrounding it. Finally, James realized that this lump was different from the others, and was persuaded (by his wife) to see me.

The lump had all the characteristics – the raised rolled pearly edge, the red colour, the small blood vessels ('telangiectasia') and the central dimple – of a basal cell cancer (BCC), or rodent ulcer. It was also in the right site, the angle between the nose and the cheek, for a classic 'rodent'. It needed to be removed, and this was a job, because of its size and position, that had to be done by a specialist. As is the rule in our area of the country, he was seen within two weeks. The operation involved removing the BCC and replacing it with a full-thickness skin graft. Radiotherapy was considered, but rejected, as the answer because of the possibility of destroying the cartilage in the centre of the nose (the nasal septum) and the slightly increased risk of a radiation-induced second cancer developing at the site. If James had been older, say in his seventies, radiation may well have been judged the treatment of choice.

James now has a tiny scar at the angle of his nose and cheek that no one, apart from a doctor, would notice. He doesn't notice it himself, but then he isn't a man to pride himself on his beauty!

Mary

Mary had reached the age of 58 without a blemish on her face. Then, out of the blue, a small spot appeared on her left cheek about a third of the way from her nose to her ear, at about the same level as the tip of her nose. At first it was no more than a pinhead in size, but over several weeks it slowly grew until it was around 3 millimetres in diameter. She described it herself as being 'punched out' of her skin. It had the shape of an irregular red ring, inside which was an underlying pink area of what looked like raw flesh. She had assumed that it was just a 'spot' that had developed after a midge bite, and that it would heal on its own. She had used an assortment of creams and ointments on it, and only when it didn't respond to them, or to the passing of time, did she decide to see me.

A close look at it revealed the same tiny group of blood vessels in the skin on and around the 'spot' – the telangiectasia also present in James's case. There was no lump: there was just this central ulcer around which was a red rim of skin. This is the classical appearance of an 'infiltrative' or 'morphoeic' BCC, so she was referred as an urgent case to the skin clinic.

The dermatologist used a method called Mohs' micrographic surgery (MMS) to remove the ulcer. This involves removing it layer by layer until all the margins of the ulcer shrink and eventually disappear. This ensures that the whole BCC is removed. It leaves, initially, a deeper hole in the face than the original BCC, which is either allowed to heal naturally over a few weeks or may be covered by a skin graft. In Mary's case it was left to heal slowly, leaving her with a tiny scar that she was easily able to cover with make-up.

Arthur

Arthur, a retired gardener in his early seventies, asked our practice nurse if she could recommend a shampoo for 'a patch of scurf' that had been bothering him for about a year. He had tried anti-dandruff shampoos and various proprietary creams, but they hadn't helped. It wasn't itchy or sore, but it did seem to be spreading, though only very slowly. The nurse wisely referred him to one of the doctors.

The 'scurf' was a red patch of scaly skin about 3 centimetres across, lying in the scalp in the hair just behind the temple. It wasn't weeping, had never caused pain or itching, and he had only asked for an opinion because his son, a nurse himself, thought it needed attention. Arthur was not unwell. He had not previously had skin trouble, something unusual for a professional gardener who had been in close contact with many plants, weedkillers and insecticides over his long career. Nor had he had any allergies.

To the doctor, the patch didn't seem like eczema, dandruff or

4

psoriasis. Eczema 'weeps' from time to time; dandruff rarely appears as a single patch, and produces a cloud of dust-like skin particles in the hair; and psoriasis in the scalp – although scaly as in Arthur's case – is usually widespread and accompanied by patches elsewhere on the skin. Arthur's doctor decided that it might be cancerous and sent him as an urgent referral to the dermatologist.

The doctor was correct in his diagnosis. The dermatologist took a small piece of tissue (a biopsy) from the 'patch' and sent it for analysis. It was reported as a 'superficial basal cell cancer'. BCCs appear in different forms. In Arthur's case there was no lump (as with James) and no ulcer (as with Mary). The affected skin was red and flat, level with the surrounding skin, and the only other abnormality is its tendency to shed scales from its centre – in fact, the symptom that worried Arthur's son and that had brought his father to the doctor.

Trying to remove surgically a patch as large as this would have left a big defect in the skin that would have been difficult to repair. Arthur was seen in 2005, the year in which for the first time an effective immune therapy was licensed in the UK for this form of BCC. Arthur was offered imiquimod (Aldara). This is a cream that is applied directly to the affected skin and to a small margin of healthy skin around it once daily for five days a week over several weeks. He was warned that the patch would 'flare up' in the first few weeks, but that the inflammation would then subside, and the skin return to normal. That is precisely what happened, much to his amazement, to that of his son and, to be honest, his GP. How imiquimod works is described later, in Chapter 6.

Jean
Jean, now in her early sixties, knocked the front of her left leg against a wooden chair when visiting a friend over the Easter holidays. Unfortunately the sharp edge of the chair caused her skin to split, leaving a small open wound, about 3 centimetres across. Having had some experience as an auxiliary nurse, Jean didn't want to bother her doctor or the practice nurse about it, so she dressed it herself. Every day she cleaned it and applied a fresh piece of Vaseline gauze to it, and she expected it to heal within a week or two.

However, by the beginning of June, the wound was not only still open and weeping a little, but it was bigger than it had been, with a red, raised, rough-looking edge all round it. In the centre was a yellow pit, from which a little thick fluid oozed each day, so that the dressing was always a little stained when she changed it. The wound was painless, and as she thought that it must be infected, she was concerned. Jean had thought from her nursing experience that infections usually cause pain, and that they are normally quickly overcome by clean dressings and routine care.

The duty doctor in the practice was concerned enough, on looking at the wound for only a few minutes, to send her for an urgent appointment at the skin clinic. In our area, that means a guaranteed appointment within two weeks, but usually the waiting time is even shorter. Jean was seen in four days.

A story of a wound caused by an accident failing to heal always raises suspicions in a GP's mind. It is not that a wound may become malignant, but that an area of skin that has become cancerous is more likely not to heal if it is injured – and is more likely to produce a bigger wound than expected of a normal patch of skin. Her GP suspected that Jean probably had an early cancer on the shin, and that knocking it resulted in a much larger area of damage than any trauma to normal skin might produce. Jean may well not have noticed that there was anything wrong with her shin until she knocked it.

This isn't always the case. Areas of very long-standing skin infections, such as leg ulcers due to varicose veins or other causes of poor circulation, such as diabetes or smoking, can produce cancers in their margins. Whether this is due to the chemical changes in the skin due to the infecting bacteria or to failure of the body's localized immune response system we still aren't sure, but it is one reason for doctors taking leg ulcers seriously and making every effort to heal them.

The angry-looking raised and lumpy edge to the ulcer and the depth to which it had eroded into the skin led the GP to think that this might be a squamous cell cancer (SCC), and this was the reason for the urgent referral. She was proved right. A piece sent to the laboratory confirmed that it was an SCC. The most appropriate treatment for an SCC is to remove it all at operation, including a wide margin of normal skin around it. The surgeon used a 'split skin' graft, taken from the front of Jean's thigh. It is enough for the moment to say that this involves taking a thin sheet of skin from the thigh and placing it over the area of healthy tissue under the skin from which the tumour has been removed; I will explain this further in the chapter on surgical treatments of cancers. The area of thigh from which the graft has been taken is left to heal normally – and in Jean's case it did so very well. She now has a patch of skin on her shin that is lighter in colour and a little different in texture from the skin around it, but she is not concerned. For her, the important news was that all the cancer had been removed and there is no reason to expect that it might return.

Robert

Robert, aged 45, had worked as a motor mechanic since he was 16. He enjoyed nothing more than messing around in engines, in his overalls, all day long. His wife understood this very well, and had taken over the paperwork for his business: she enjoyed the responsibility, he enjoyed the freedom from office work, and the business thrived. They made a good team, serving the local farming community.

Then one day in the shower after work, Robert noticed a small lump in the middle of the right side of the skin of his scrotum next to where it rested against his thigh. At first he thought that it might be a small cyst or even an insect bite (it was high summer and biting insects were common around the garage, which was on the edge of the village, near some woods by a river). After a week or so it had the feel, and the size, of a small pea, rising up out of the skin. Robert still felt that this was nothing to worry about, as it wasn't painful and he felt perfectly well. It was only after around a month, when it was beginning to make him feel uncomfortable – it was catching on the edge of his Y-fronts – that he thought he should make an appointment to see me.

The lump had by this time developed a small 'pit' in the centre, which was firm and yellowish. There was one small area that had a fleshy lump within it, like a tiny cauliflower. When I felt the scrotum, the lump was fixed into it – I couldn't move it around free of the overlying skin. Nor could I really define a smooth edge to it – it seemed to merge in an irregular way with the healthy skin around it, which was thicker than the rest of his scrotum.

Added to that ominous sign, I didn't like the way the lump felt so hard. It was close to the 'feel' of a stone, with no 'give' in it, as it might have had, had it been a cyst, say, full of fluid or sweat secretions. This suggested a malignancy, especially as it was painless. I would have been happier if Robert had winced as I examined the lump, as this would suggest infection. Finally, I placed a pen-torch behind the lump and switched it on. The light didn't pass through it: it had a dark shadow, strongly suggesting solid tissue and not a cyst. It was clearly something I had to refer with urgency to the skin clinic.

We have known about skin cancers like this since the eighteenth century, when the great surgeon of the day, Percival Pott, described cancers of the scrotum in chimneysweeps. Soot and oils from chimneys would collect in the crotch of their trousers and their constant contact with the skin of the scrotum led to the cancer. Motor mechanics whose working clothes are often permeated with oil still face that risk. Industrial oils and skin don't mix well together.

Happily, Robert had come to me in time. The squamous cell cancer he had developed hadn't spread beyond the scrotum, and it was eradicated surgically without the need to remove a testicle. If it had spread beyond the scrotal skin towards the testicle and the groin, it could have led to a much more drastic operation.

George

I was reminded of Robert's case about a year later, when George, a 48-year-old fisherman, asked about a 'spot' that had grown on the back of his right hand. It had grown much faster than Robert's tumour, reaching more than 1 centimetre in diameter in around four weeks. George hadn't come to me sooner because he thought the spot was the result of an infection caught when gutting fish on board the boat, and that it would settle on its own. He was away from home for weeks at a time, so this was his first opportunity to see me.

At first sight I feared the worst: the 'spot' looked almost exactly like Robert's tumour. It was dome-shaped, with a firm, thickened rounded edge, in the centre of which was a depression with something black in the middle of it. I used a tiny spoon-like instrument to probe that central area, and was relieved to be able to lift a piece of thick, mushy brown material out of it. This was a substance called keratin, the material that forms the outer layer of skin, and it showed me that the tumour was a 'kerato-acanthoma'.

Kerato-acanthomas are a halfway house between an overgrowth of normal skin and a cancer. They form on sun-exposed areas of skin, so they are presumably a reaction to repeated sunburn. They typically arise out of the blue on the back of a hand or on the cheeks, and grow very fast – faster than Robert's squamous cell tumour. They can reach 2 centimetres in diameter in around two months, and then they seem to 'run out of steam'. If left to themselves, they stop growing and remain at that size for a further two months, before shrinking away, leaving an unsightly scar behind.

In the past, George's tumour would have been left to run its course, but we don't do that today. Because there is always a chance that a part of a kerato-acanthoma might harbour malignant squamous cancer cells, GPs faced with one now send the patient to the skin clinic, where the specialist will remove it surgically and stitch the wound carefully together, leaving as little scarring as possible.

In fact, when the pathologist examined the material that had been removed from George's hand she found a small area of squamous cell cancer in its margins. Happily, it had been entirely removed, and George now has an additional tiny scar on his hand to complement all the others he inflicted on himself when gutting fish. There has been no recurrence of the cancer in the ten years since he had it removed.

Fred

Fred grows chrysanthemums and carnations. Not just a few – over the years he must have sold millions of them to garden centres and nurseries. He was just 41 when he asked me to look at his skin. It wasn't easy to see at first glance the cause of his anxiety. He had a ruddy complexion from years of working in his greenhouses and fields, but the colour of his skin wasn't his concern. Nor were his numerous freckles: he had had them since he was a boy, and they hadn't changed. He explained that, with his fair hair and his light-blue eyes, he had always been sensitive to the sun, so that he had worn a hat most of the time when he was outside. Though in his younger days, when he had more hair, Fred had often forgotten to put it on.

He wasn't sure if he was wasting my time, but he had noticed recently that the skin on the right side of his forehead, close to the temple, on the back of his hands and forearms, and the bald patch at the front of his head, 'felt as if it had lots of tiny hard bits in it'.

A closer look at his skin, and particularly how it felt when I brushed my fingertips over it, gave the explanation. He had multiple 'solar keratoses'. They are small areas of scaly roughness in the skin, like tiny seeds, that appear after years of exposure to the sun. The paler the skin is and the more intense the sunshine, the faster and the more extensive are the patches of keratoses.

He had so many that it would have been impractical to try to remove them surgically, but I had to do something, because a small number of these areas of sun damage can change into squamous cell cancers. It was best for a specialist to decide on how to treat them. He had a wide choice, the details of which are given in the chapter on therapy, but the possible treatments included cauterization, freezing or a cream containing 5-fluorouracil. The dermatologist opted for the last: it is an anti-cancer agent that is absorbed by the abnormal cells and then destroys them. Fred was advised first to wash and dry the affected areas, then to put the cream on them twice a day for six weeks. He was told that the skin would become red and sore soon after starting the treatment, but that he should continue to use it. After the six weeks, he might be able to use an antibiotic cream to ease any residual infection, which can be a side-effect of the treatment. He was told that the keratoses should heal with no scar – and that's what happened.

He has used sunblock, long-sleeved shirts and a floppy hat from then on, and hasn't looked back. His sons have joined him in the business, and he has warned them about over-exposure to the sun (they are all fair-haired and freckled like him). He spends more time in the office, managing his ever-expanding business, and when he takes a break, he sits in the shade.

Angela
Angela, a secondary school teacher, was 51 when she first noticed

something wrong in the skin of her upper right arm, just below the shoulder. She had had eczema as a child, and her daughter, now 22, had also had it from the time she was a toddler until she started her periods at 12. Angela not unnaturally thought, from this personal history, that this was another patch of eczema connected with the hormone changes of the menopause. She didn't want any fuss, so she simply bought some hydrocortisone cream from the pharmacy and treated herself. She knew from experience that it would eventually respond to the steroid hormone.

She was surprised that it didn't disappear fairly quickly, but it still didn't bother her much, as it wasn't itchy. Even when it spread a little beyond the original patch, she wasn't concerned about it. That lack of concern was reinforced by a well-meaning friend who, noticing the slight scaliness in the centre of the growing 'spot' and its bright-red colour, suggested that it was a patch of psoriasis. Angela had known another friend with psoriasis, and was aware that it was a benign skin disease likely to disappear of its own accord, so she still didn't ask her GP's advice. Instead she bought some anti-psoriasis cream from the pharmacist, and tried that.

It made no difference. In fact, the patch enlarged further. It had a very well-defined edge that marked it out from the surrounding skin, but it was very irregular in outline – she described it aptly as looking like a map of an island with fjords and bays and inlets. Taking the geographic analogy further, she said there were now small lumps in it, like a relief map of rolling hills.

I was amused by her schoolmistress's approach to her skin problem, but not by the lesion itself. She had Bowen's disease, which is the name for a change towards cancer within skin cells. The technical name for this type of change is intra-epidermal carcinoma or carcinoma-in-situ. Under the microscope, the cells in such a patch look like squamous cancer cells, but they have not yet developed the ability to spread beyond that area of skin to distant organs. Quite large areas of skin can become affected by Bowen's disease: in Angela's case, it was a roughly circular patch of about 3 centimetres in diameter by the time she came to see me – by this time, she was 53. Two years had passed between her first noticing it and coming to get a medical opinion.

It is quite common for people with Bowen's disease to wait for a year or two before they seek help. They are shocked when they find that they have delayed so long with a potentially lethal condition, although dermatologists take great pains to reassure them that very few cases do eventually become overtly cancerous and life threatening. In Angela's case, the dermatologist was very understanding. He took a small biopsy that confirmed the diagnosis and explained that he would use a combination of treatments on it, including the 5-fluorouracil that was so helpful with Fred's keratoses. If it responded well to the cream, that might be all that was necessary, but Angela would need regular check-ups to make sure that any change for the worse would be caught in time.

Catherine

When Catherine was four years old, her parents emigrated from Britain to Brisbane. They lived in Australia for ten years before they returned for family reasons. Catherine was a sun-loving girl, and spent as much of her time at the beach as she could. She grew up with the Australian warnings about sunburn on fair skin, so she knew about wearing a floppy hat and long-sleeved shirts, and using suncreams. I met her when she was 28, some 14 years after coming home to the UK, and for a while I had no idea that she had spent so much of her childhood in a near-tropical climate.

So when she asked about a spot on her back that Hugh, her husband, had noticed, I wasn't too troubled by her story – until I saw the spot, that is. It was what many people would call a 'mole'. It was a round black disc with a darker spot in the middle and different shades, ranging from brown to blue to black, over its surface. In places it was flat against the skin; in others it was raised a millimetre or so. Its edges faded into the skin around it, so that it appeared that there was some pigment under the surface surrounding the main patch. Catherine's husband, who came with her, said that he thought that it had grown recently, both upwards, so that it projected further out from the flat skin around it, and outwards, so that the disc was enlarging.

Catherine felt nothing untoward and was generally well, but both she and Hugh were rightly worried that it might be a melanoma. I had the same worry. I phoned our dermatologist and explained the possibilities, and it was arranged for Catherine to be seen at the next clinic. The dermatologist examined it, together with her colleague, a plastic surgeon, and they concluded that it should be removed in its entirety at the clinic, in a 'one-stop' procedure. The microscope confirmed that it was a melanoma, and Catherine started on a long road of investigations. Thankfully, there was no detectable spread to other sites in her body, but she is not yet in the clear. At the time of writing, she has been recurrence-free for four years. As each year passes she has a better chance of avoiding the return of the melanoma. She is happy to remain in the UK and stay away from strong sunshine. It is a small inconvenience, she says, if it is going to save her life.

Whether that is true or not is still a debate among the experts. The arguments for and against the proposal that melanoma is caused by excess exposure to the sun are explained in Chapter 3. In the meantime, Catherine, Hugh and their two children take their holidays roaming the Scottish Highlands, and they love it. They are all fair-skinned and freckled, so they don't consider spending summer holidays in the heat of the Mediterranean. They are still wary of the sun: even in the Hebrides, the long days of midsummer (the sun can shine for nearly 20 hours a day) can leave you with sunburn, so they take sunblock with them, and enjoy fishing, walking, golfing and the magic hospitality of the islanders. It's a choice that I can appreciate.

Gillian
Gillian prided herself on her tan. She was a slim young woman who liked to look brown all year round, so she visited the gym every week for a workout and a session on a sunbed to keep herself in shape and to 'top up' her tan. She was fortunate enough to be able to take two holidays a year, in which she indulged herself on a beach – first in the south of Spain where she and her husband had a timeshare, and then in the winter, usually in Goa or the Maldives, with an occasional break in Thailand. Gillian reasoned that as she tanned easily and had a naturally brown skin, she didn't need to use sunblocks. As long as she didn't burn, she thought, she was protected against the dangers of the sun.

I wish she had been right. At the age of 31, she noticed that a small brown spot on her shoulder – she called it a mole – had enlarged and darkened, so that it was now almost black. Gillian had quite a few similar moles on her body and legs, but she had never taken much notice of them. However, this one stood out when she was wearing an off-the-shoulder top, and that wouldn't do. And she didn't like the second 'mole' that had appeared near it, like a spoke from the hub of the first one.

I didn't like it either. I was fairly certain that she had two melanomas, the second arising probably under the skin from the first. She also had a small firm lump at the base of her neck, in the triangle between her collarbone and the muscles that ran between her neck and her shoulder. This could well be a swollen lymph gland, and might well be a spread from the skin into the deeper tissues. The next step was to examine her thoroughly, which began to alarm her.

There was little I could do to reassure her. Her liver was enlarged, and there were other ominous lumps in her abdomen and in her armpits. She had to be admitted to our specialist oncology (cancer) unit as a probable case of melanoma with spread to other organs.

Gillian, tragically, was one of the people we could not save. She was another statistic in the toll that melanoma takes in the UK today – a figure nearly ten times higher than it was 30 years ago. In spite of everything the specialists tried, Gillian died within a few months, a terrible loss at such an early age.

Why people like Gillian develop such a lethal type of melanoma is still unknown. As I have already said, the debate about whether or not exposing the skin to too much sun induces cancer is still being waged – although it must be admitted that the vast majority of the experts believe that too much sun *can* stimulate skin cancers in fair-skinned people. (I have devoted Chapter 3 to examining the arguments put forward by both sides.) Whether Gillian's devotion to getting a tan had brought her particular cancer to its lethal state we will never know, but it does seem, in retrospect, that if you have many 'moles' on your body, it is better not to risk a sun-induced change in them. About a quarter of malignant melanomas start in pre-existing moles – but that means that three-quarters of them arise out of the blue, in previously normal skin. Most people have several 'moles' that remain benign – the same size and colour with no potential for spread – and if they are all taken into account, their chances of becoming malignant are around one in a million.

William

Like Gillian, William has 'moles' on his skin. At the last count there were nearly 200 of them on his back, his chest and tummy. They were not raised above the skin, but flat within it, either round or oval in shape with smooth edges demarcating them from the surrounding skin. They varied from 1–2 millimetres to 1 centimetre across, and were a uniform brown colour. Medically, they are called 'pigmented naevi'.

Unlike Gillian, William was only too aware of what the moles might mean. His mother and her father, his grandfather, had also had hundreds of naevi. His grandfather, a sailor, had developed a melanoma in one of them and had died in his forties, leaving a widow and young daughter. William's mother, Margaret, had heard that her father's father, William's great-grandfather, and an uncle had also died of melanoma, but she had no written evidence for the story, as they had died before she was born. Margaret knew only too well that the moles on her own back could follow her father's example. Over the years she had taken great pains, even using two large mirrors in her bedroom to see better, to make sure that the moles did not make the change from benign mole to malignant melanoma. When Margaret married, she asked her husband to carry on the examinations. He even photographed her back as a reference point for any future change.

Intuitively, because it was in the days before doctors had made the link between the sun and cancer, Margaret kept out of the sun, and she warned William, from a very young age, to do the same.

Margaret did develop melanoma, but not in one of the moles on her back. She noticed a change in size and shape in a mole on her chest, just above her left breast. It had darkened, too. She took her worries about it to her doctor, and the mole was removed. Unlike her father, Margaret survived, and now, well into her sixties, she remains healthy. She still examines her skin regularly, as she knows that she has a higher than normal chance, after one melanoma, of developing another.

When he was 18, knowing about the melanomas in both his mother and grandfather, William asked his doctor about his melanoma risk. With at least two, and possibly more than three, cases of melanoma in his immediate family, he was told that he was at high risk – perhaps as much as 30 times higher than normal. William decided to follow his mother's example, and keep a watch on his skin. His father has photographed William's skin, back and front, as a reference.

So far, William, now in his early thirties, has not noticed a change in his naevi. He keeps out of the sun, and his wife has brown eyes, dark hair, and a skin that tans easily with only three or four 'moles'. Their two children are lucky to have escaped William's skin problem: their skins are like their mother's, which is a source of great relief to the couple.

William and Margaret are unusual, in that their skin problem accounts for only around 2 per cent of all cases of melanoma. They have almost certainly inherited a gene that fails to protect their skin from the damage caused by the sun's ultraviolet rays, and that interferes with the skin's natural defences against the initiation and spread of cancer within it. The mechanisms behind this are explained in Chapter 7.

A warning here. If you have a lot of pigmented moles on your back, but there has been no melanoma in your close family, don't assume that you are at as much risk as William and Margaret. Their risk was a combination of a strongly positive family history and the moles. Without the evidence of relatives with melanoma, your risk is very much lower than theirs – but it is not zero. Do look at your skin regularly and become familiar with your spots. Only then will you know when one has changed. Chapter 6 goes into this in much more detail.

Peter
Peter, a businessman in his late fifties, had the same illness as the actor Paul Eddington, famous for sit-coms such as *The Good Life* and *Yes Minister*. It started with a few patches of what were first thought to be eczema – areas of red skin that itched and occasionally oozed a little fluid. Over several years, despite various creams and ointments, the small patches became larger, to form what doctors call 'plaques' – flat areas of abnormal skin that look and feel firmer than the normal skin around them. As the

skin failed to heal, Peter's doctor sent him for further investigations. The specialist found enlarged lymph nodes near the affected skin, and small lumps in the skin itself. He recognized it as early 'mycosis fungoides', a form of lymphoma, or cancer of the white cells called T-lymphocytes. Over the next four years, and more than 20 years after he had noticed the patch, Peter underwent a series of treatments, involving anti-cancer ointments, radiotherapy, ultraviolet light and chemotherapy by mouth. It has kept the condition at bay for several years, but in the long term we still have no cure. Peter is now in the later stages of his mycosis fungoides, but still holds out hope that research will provide yet another way of helping him.

Sadly, Paul Eddington died from his illness, but before he did so, in a most moving programme, he thanked the doctors doing research into skin cancers like his, asking the public to continue to support them.

2

The healthy skin

Having bought or borrowed this book, you presumably have skin cancer yourself, or are caring for someone with it. Reading the first chapter may have opened your eyes to the different forms that skin cancer takes, and you will probably have found one case history that mirrors yours or that of the person you care for. This chapter describes the structure of the skin and the cells within it that can become cancerous. Knowing from which cell type a cancer has started tells your oncologist (cancer specialist) what to expect in the way of malignancy and possible spread and, most important, how to treat it with the highest chance of success.

Your skin has two fundamental layers, the epidermis (the outside layer) and the dermis (the layer just underneath it). The epidermis ranges from 0.07 to 0.12 millimetres in thickness, being thickest on the soles of the feet, and only slightly less thick on the palms of the hands and fingers. If your work involves constant rubbing and pressure, the epidermis thickens much more. That explains calluses on the hands of oarsmen or golfers, or people who handle heavy machinery for hours at a time. The dermis is on average 1–2 millimetres thick on most of the body, being a little thinner on the eyelids and thicker on the palms and soles.

Cut your skin so that it bleeds, and you have cut entirely through the epidermis and dermis, to expose the sub-dermal tissues underneath. Just shave off the upper surface, the outer 'hornified' epidermal layer (as in paring a corn or verruca), and it will grow again without a scar. Take away the full thickness of the skin (that is, the dermis and epidermis) and you will be left with a scar, although after a time you may not see it. Normal skin is excellent at self-repair.

The dermis and epidermis meet in a very well-defined junction called the basal layer, which is in effect your skin factory. The basal cells in this layer are the factory production line, with the cells of the epidermis being their end-product. They start as a layer of cubical cells that flatten to become the squamous cells (squamous means a scale, as in fish skin, or pavement-like). Each new squamous cell pushes its predecessor further outwards from the basal layer, and therefore further from the source of its nutrition, the circulation beneath. The epidermis contains no blood vessels, so that eventually the older squamous cells die from lack of nutrition, leaving an outer 'carpet' of dead remnants of cells that are interlocked and made up of keratin, a tough waterproof material. We were taught at medical school that keratin is vital if we want to go out in the rain: if we were not covered in it, we would soak up the water, swell up and burst. It also prevents the underlying tissues from drying out, so that if we didn't have that keratin covering, we would shrivel up in dry weather.

The keratin surface flakes away ('desquamates', or de-scales) with normal everyday life. You see desquamation every time you clean your bath. Wash your body in bathwater and you leave behind the outermost layer of epidermis as a thin discolouration on the sides of the bath. The more active the desquamation (the faster you wear the skin away), the more active is the basal cell layer in producing more squamous cells to replace those that are lost.

We can take the factory analogy further. If the basal cells are our employees on the production line and the squamous cells the product, we also need sensors to detect problems, air-conditioning to keep the factory conditions right for optimum production, and protection against changes in climate that might damage the factory. Our skin has all of these – and they can all go wrong.

The sensors are the nerve endings that detect heat and cold, touch and pain, and position in space. When the hot or cold sensors 'fire off', we react automatically by closing down the circulation in the dermis to preserve body heat in the cold and opening it to get rid of waste heat when we are too warm. We react to touch and pain with the appropriate muscle responses and the 'space' detectors work with the brain to keep us well balanced. If the sun is too fierce, 'melanocytes', cells in the basal layer that produce the pigment melanin, switch on to give us a tan. People from tropical countries are naturally darker than those from northern Europe because they have more melanocytes, which are in constant production, and are the equivalent of the factory 'blinds'.

The air-conditioning? That comes from the combined work of sweat glands and hair follicles. When it's too hot, the sweat glands produce salty fluid that evaporates from the surface. As it does so, it takes heat of evaporation (remember your school physics?) with it, cooling the skin and our bodies. And although with evolution we have lost most of our body hair, we still have the remnants of another body temperature-regulating system in the form of 'goose-pimples'. Each goosepimple is the base of a tiny hair. Our ancestors were presumably covered in what amounts to fur: thick hair that 'stood up' when it was cold to give us a thick layer of insulation. On warmer days it would lie flat. Goosepimples are the result of the muscles at the base of each hair contracting to try to make it 'stand up'. Our hair is so sparse that it is no longer effective, but it is a reminder that we did have an effective way of keeping warm before we had clothes.

Skin is also our first line of defence against infections, irritants and allergens (such as certain plant juices and chemicals), so the dermis is full of small blood vessels that can provide at short notice the white blood cells and the range of chemical substances in the blood plasma that we need to tackle them. In the sub-dermal tissues around these vessels there are also tissue white cells, such as specialized lymphocytes, that come to our rescue when our defences are compromised.

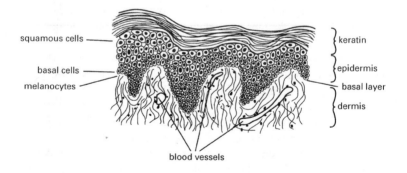

Figure 1 The appearance of normal skin
as seen through a microscope

By now you will appreciate that the skin is a very active organ. The dermis and epidermis are very active tissues with a high turnover of cells with very specific jobs to do. Normally these jobs are done perfectly: occasionally they go wrong, though, and that can mean the development of cancer.

Cancer arises from a particular type of cell. Therefore a basal cell gives a basal cell cancer, a squamous cell produces a squamous cell cancer, and a melanocyte can become a melanoma. The lymphocytes in the dermis can give rise to mycosis fungoides, as in the case of Peter in the case history in the last chapter. There are even very rare tumours of the sweat glands and the hair follicles, but because they are very slow-growing cells they are almost always benign. In my many years in practice I have never seen anyone with a sweat gland or hair follicle cancer, but sadly all the other types of skin cancer are relatively common. So common, in fact, that in the UK and other European countries they have overtaken all other cancers in the tumour league tables.

Why this should be is a matter of discussion among the specialists: some of the experts suggest changes in the environment are the cause; others point to much higher rates of sunburn in holidaymakers. Still others suggest that it is just a natural feature of a population in which a much higher proportion than ever before have reached old age.

Chapter 3 summarizes the debate that is still raging (I use the word advisedly) among the researchers on why skin cancer is so common, and what the media (which I suppose includes this book) should do to help people avoid it.

3

The doctors' messages to the public – are they correct?

The most effective way to reduce your risk of developing cancer is to avoid the circumstances that promote it, but for cancer in general that may not be easy. To begin with, you may have a genetic predisposition to skin cancer, and the only way to alter that would be to choose different parents, and it is too late for that.

However, if the cancer is the result of something in the environment or the way you live, then these factors can be avoided or changed. Fifty years ago, the link between smoking and rising rates of death from lung cancer was proven beyond doubt to the medical profession. It took most of that half-century, though, for the public and the politicians to realize fully the wreckage that tobacco wreaked on lives. Thankfully, at last the authorities in several countries (Ireland, Canada, Scotland and Norway among them) have banned smoking from most public places, and even England has finally changed the law.

The message about sunburn and skin cancer emerged in the 1970s, mainly from Australia, but it was taken up in the UK by Professor Rona MacKie, in Glasgow, who reported a steep rise in skin cancers among Scots who had taken regular holidays abroad and used sunbeds. The Australian authorities were the first to take the message seriously, which is not surprising, as around one in ten Australians of European descent was developing skin cancer. Their advice to wear a hat with a wide brim and shirts with sleeves, to use sunblocking creams or sunscreens and to sit in the shade rather than the sun has started to lower their skin cancer rates.

With Europe's anti-sunburn campaigns starting two decades later than Australia's, the figures here are still rising. But even Europeans who live around the Mediterranean coast don't have the same sun exposure as the Australians of Brisbane, Cairns or Darwin, so should we bother? The answer to that question is not so clear cut as it might seem.

In 1992 the International Association for Research into Cancer

(IARC) published a volume entitled *IARC Monographs on the Evaluation of Carcinogenic Risks to Humans: Solar and Ultraviolet Radiation, Volume 55.* It confirmed to its readers (there were probably very few, but they were opinion leaders in the medical profession) that 'ultraviolet exposure from the sun is a major cause of melanoma and other skin cancers'. Consequently, the bombardment of the public with messages about the dangers of the sun started from that year. Most of us have heard them:

1 Avoid the sun.
2 No tan is a healthy tan.
3 Your lifetime risk of any skin cancer is 1 in 5.
4 Your lifetime risk of a melanoma is 1 in 74.
5 It is only childhood sunburn that really matters. You are most exposed to the sun, and to being burnt by it, when you are a child, and this is the time when the cancer process is most likely to be initiated.
6 Don't rely on sunscreens to protect you.

Let's look at these one at a time:

Message 1 – avoid the sun

If the sun is the cause of our rising numbers of cases of skin cancer, then it would seem that 'avoid the sun' is a simple solution. Of course, this advice is ignored. We northern Europeans take every opportunity to sunbathe in the summer, because we rarely get the chance to do it and it feels so good. We feel the better for it, provided that we don't burn. In fact, it is so popular to sunbathe that the message has changed subtly over the years from 'avoid the sun' to 'limit the time you spend in the sun'. That seems sensible, but is it, in reality?

Dermatologist and oncologist Dr Martin Weinstock of Brown University in Providence, Rhode Island, USA, has his doubts. He raises the question of what you should do instead. If you are avoiding the sun, do you take less exercise than you would if you were enjoying a good summer day outside? If you are exerting yourself less, then you face an increased risk of heart disease, diabetes, high blood pressure, colon cancer, depression, obesity and early death. 'Together', he writes, 'these outweigh skin cancer in overall impact on health' (Weinstock, 2004). He adds that 'we need Vitamin D for healthy bones and muscles. A major source of Vitamin D is from the action of sunlight on our skin: the more we expose our skin to the sun, the more Vitamin D we make. Vitamin D levels in the general public are often less than they should be, and reducing sun exposure may make this worse.'

I'm not sure about this last statement. If Vitamin D levels really are so low, then we should be seeing many more cases than we do of rickets, the bone-stunting and bone-bending disease that used to be so common in Victorian Britain in very poor children. In fact, in my whole life as a GP I have never had to deal with a case of rickets caused by Vitamin D deficiency – and nor have any of the GP colleagues whom I have asked about it.

However, let's for the moment take Dr Weinstock's comment as accurate. We can easily take extra Vitamin D by eating the correct foods or by swallowing a supplement every day, but very few of us are willing to change our lifelong eating habits or to take a daily pill when we don't feel a direct or immediate benefit from it. If we doctors still want to exhort people to avoid the sun, then we should be equally emphatic about taking in more Vitamin D in the form of food or as a supplement.

How did we develop a skin that makes Vitamin D in the first place? The darker your skin is (that is, if you originate from countries near the Equator, such as Central Africa or the South Asian subcontinent), the less Vitamin D your skin makes when you emigrate to European countries. In your country of origin, there is more than enough hot sun all the year round to keep up your Vitamin D levels. It seems, however, that when early man left Africa for Europe he had to reduce his ability to make melanin so as to increase his Vitamin D-forming capacity. We developed a lighter skin in order to keep up our Vitamin D levels. So is it absolutely wise to keep out of the sun now?

Some dermatologists would say that it was. At a 2005 dermatology seminar for GPs in the UK, the lecturer proposed that no one should spend more than five minutes a day in the sun, and no minutes at all at midday in the summer. More than that, and the person would have an unacceptable risk of developing melanoma.

Admittedly this was extreme even for a dermatologist whose life is devoted to curing skin cancer. The times were an estimate, not taken from studies of people with measured different exposures to sunshine over many years, but from recall by patients of episodes of sunburn as a child, and assuming that allowing your skin to redden or burn increases melanoma risk. In fact, although numbers of cases of skin cancers are rising, we do not know for sure that sunbathing to excess is their direct cause.

What we do know is that fair-skinned people who live near the Equator have high rates of malignant melanoma, most of the cases being in Australia and New Zealand. Dark-skinned people have much lower rates of melanoma than the fair-skinned. In people with fair skin, melanomas do arise mainly where the skin has been repeatedly exposed to the sun, such as the hands, arms, face and scalp. The soles of the feet are the main risk area for melanoma in darker-skinned people.

You can conclude from this that fair-skinned people should avoid excess exposure to the sun, but that this is less important for those with darker skins. The problem is – how much exposure is too much? The figures from the Antipodes clearly show that people of European background who move to Australia or the North Island of New Zealand should follow the rules and protect themselves from the sun. Should the British do the same?

The facts suggest that we should certainly avoid sunburn, as it may cause changes that could lead to cancers in years to come. The midday sun on a summer holiday in Italy, Greece or Spain can be as damaging as that in Australia. But what about other times and places? That's where the debate gets as hot as the beach.

Dr Malcolm Kendrick, a GP in the UK, wrote in July 2005 in *Pulse* (a journal for doctors) on the subject. He agreed with Dr Weinstock that the sun may in fact be good for you. He quotes W. B. Grant in the journal *Cancer* (Grant, 2002). Dr Grant compared sun exposure to cancer rates throughout the USA, and found that 'solar UVB radiation is associated with reduced risk of cancer of the breast, colon, ovary and prostate as well as non-Hodgkin's lymphoma'. According to Dr Grant, the US states with the highest exposure to the sun had the lowest rates of these cancers. He added that the risks of bladder, oesophageal, kidney, lung, pancreatic, rectal, stomach and uterine cancers were also lower in those states with higher ultraviolet exposure. He was even able to calculate from his figures that each year lack of sun exposure had led to 21,700 premature deaths from cancer in Americans of European descent, 1,400 in African Americans, and 500 in Asian Americans. These are much higher figures than the 8,000 annual deaths from melanoma, many of which are on skin that the sun does not reach.

There is more. Lack of sunshine has also been implicated in rising risks of multiple sclerosis, rheumatoid arthritis, inflammatory bowel diseases such as Crohn's disease and ulcerative colitis, and even Type 1 diabetes (Cantorna and Mahon, 2004).

How can sunlight make such a difference, and be so beneficial? Dr Kendrick is sure that Vitamin D is the key. For most of the twentieth century we thought that its only function was to strengthen bone: Vitamin D pushes calcium and phosphate into bone, providing its strength. By 2005, the researchers had gathered solid evidence that it initiates the 'suicide' death of cells that have started to become cancerous – a process called apoptosis. It also helps to prevent new blood vessels forming around cancers – that is, the way that cancer cells spread to other tissues and produce the metastases mentioned in Chapter 1 (Giovannucci, 2005).

Dr Kendrick goes against all the current thinking, however, when he claims that Vitamin D is so good at prevention of cancer that 'a decent amount of sun exposure actually reduces the risk of malignant melanoma'. 'If you go outside', he writes, 'and build up a tan you will reduce the risk of all types of cancer, including melanoma.' He bases this thinking on reports that people regularly exposed to ultraviolet radiation in their occupations have a lower than average risk of developing this form of cancer (Berwick and colleagues, 2005).

This is where I part company with Dr Kendrick. However, for the last ten years the public has been bombarded by advice that tanning is dangerous. That message is too simple, and is open to misinterpretation, and the medical profession as a whole has been guilty of promoting it in a way that can make people feel guilty about lying in the sun. That is surely wrong.

Message 2 – no tan is a healthy tan

If we have naturally pale skin, we are at higher risk of developing melanomas and other skin cancers than if we have naturally brown skin. That is a fact of life that we can't avoid. Pale-skinned people are going to develop more skin cancers than brown- or black-skinned people whether they sunbathe or not. So there is an argument, like the one put forward by Dr Kendrick, that if you start with pale skin and gently tan yourself so that your skin becomes brown, you will tend to prevent skin cancers rather than promote them.

As is often the case in medical matters, the truth is not so simple. In the process of tanning pale-coloured skin by exposing it to ultraviolet light (the wavelength of light from the sun's spectrum that stimulates the melanocytes to produce melanin), you are doing two things: you are producing more melanin, and therefore making your skin brown; and you are damaging the cells in the skin in a direction that may lead to cancer. People with pale skin who tan easily after only a short time in the sun, without going red and blistering, are at lower risk of this damage, and are less likely to develop a cancer. Those who burn easily and produce very little in the way of a tan are at much higher risk. They go red, blister, then peel, and only become a little browner after longer exposure and a lot of effort. In their case, the eventual mild tan is a sign that they have been overdoing it and inviting serious damage to their skin.

So the idea that all tans are unhealthy is misleading. Today's lifestyles mean that most of the time we hide our skins from the sun. Even if we have a naturally brown skin, the colour may fade during the months we are working, but it returns again when we make for the sun on our holidays. If you are in that category, then a gentle tan on holiday is only returning your skin to its natural state, and there's little evidence that it will cause any harm.

However, if you are fair-haired and have blue eyes, with pale skin and freckles, and with 'moles' dotted around your body, tanning is not for you. It is better to stay your natural colour. In fact, I would replace the 'no tan is a healthy tan' message with this one: 'the healthiest colour for your skin is the colour you were born with'. That's correct for all ethnic groups and people with all types of skin colour, and it still lets people understand that trying to change your skin colour by lying in the sun can be dangerous.

Just how dangerous is given by one startling statistic: the proportion of the population that now develops melanoma, the most malignant type of skin cancer, is 2,000 per cent higher than 60 years ago (Heston and colleagues, 1986; Polednak, 2001). This huge rise cannot be explained away by the suggestion that doctors are more efficient in diagnosing it: we knew as much about diagnosing melanoma in the mid-twentieth century as we do now. It is directly related to people with skin unsuitable for tanning pursuing a more brown skin on beaches and sunbeds. The 'keep the colour you were born with' message is also one that we are more likely to heed – it is a positive one, suggesting that 'good' behaviour will protect us – than the old message that equates to 'tan and you will regret it', which we react against because it induces a sense of guilt or even shame. Messages like this rarely work.

Messages 3 and 4 – you have a 1 in 7 risk of skin cancer and a 1 in 74 risk of melanoma

That 2,000 per cent rise in melanoma rates sounds horrific, and for the families afflicted by it, it can be a tragedy. But it is difficult to work out what our own risk is, over each of our lifetimes, of developing a skin cancer. Let's refer again to Dr Weinstock, who is an expert in assessing risk.

Doctors are fond of quoting 'lifetime risk' of different cancers. That is, the risk you face of a particular type of cancer from the day you were born until you die. It sounds a useful concept, but it is not as straightforward as it seems. The researchers calculate lifetime risk from the death certificates of people who have died in the years just before you were born. So for a baby born in the year 1935, his or her lifetime risk of developing melanoma was at that time 1 chance in 1,500, as calculated from the numbers of melanomas written on death certificates. Some 63 years later, in 1998, the actual risk (taken from the numbers of cases of melanoma that had actually developed until that time in babies born in 1935) was 1 in 124 for the boys and 1 in 156 for the girls – ten times the calculated lifetime risk. That figure is bound to worsen further as the survivors reached their later sixties and seventies.

For babies born in 2000, the calculated lifetime risk had risen further to 1 in 74, but it is expected that their actual risk will be ten times that – Dr Weinstock estimates it to be around 1 in 7. In other words, if rates of melanoma continue to increase as they have done in the last 50 years, people born in 2000 have a 1 in 7 chance of developing a melanoma at some time during their lives. These are close to the figures already reported in people of European origin living in Australia. Dr Weinstock sees the rise in skin cancers continuing, and blames it on changing patterns of sun exposure and artificial tans that may or may not be offset by sunscreen use and other forms of protection from the sun's rays.

So the 1 in 7 risk of skin cancer is probably accurate: the 1 in 74 risk of melanoma is probably a severe underestimate of the numbers we can expect in the mid-twenty-first century. The message to look after your skin isn't just for us – it is also for our children and grandchildren.

Message 5 – it's only childhood sunburn that really matters

Time and again, we read that what really matters as a cause of eventual skin cancer is getting sunburnt as a child. That's the time, the message goes, that the skin is most susceptible to the type of damage by the sun that can lead to cancerous changes. The cancers may take many years to arise, but the initial stimulus occurs in childhood. If that message were true, then it would give a green light for adults to lie in the sun with impunity.

Unfortunately, it isn't true.

It *is* true that when children with pale skins move to sunnier countries and are burnt by the sun, they are at higher risk of skin cancer later on. At least three studies have confirmed that migrants from temperate to hot countries are at much higher risk of melanoma in early adult life than they would have been if they had stayed at home (Holman and Armstrong, 1984; Khlat and colleagues, 1992; Swerdlow and colleagues, 1995).

However, that doesn't let adults off the hook. By 1998, the Melanoma Co-Operative Group of the European Organization for Research and Treatment of Cancer examined how sun exposure in children and adults influenced the risk of later melanoma. The adults were just as vulnerable as the children. The conclusion was that we should still protect children from over-exposure to the sun, but adults should be given similar advice.

Another myth was proven wrong in 2004. We were often told that 80 per cent of our lifetime's exposure to the sun happens when we are children. Children, the story went, spent much more time playing outdoors and children's clothes left their skin more open to the sun that the clothes of adults, whose working lives left them little time for relaxation outside. There is doubt that this was ever true, but if it was, it certainly isn't now. In 2004, Dr L. Thieden (Thieden and colleagues, 2004) strapped instruments that measured 'doses' of sunlight onto children, teenagers and adults, and found that the three groups spent similar times in the sun. Patterns of sunbathing and outdoor living that begin in childhood continue throughout our adult lives. It seems that we have a similar chance of becoming sunburnt at any time in our lives. We can't drop our guard at any age if we have the type of skin that is susceptible to a cancerous change.

Message 6 – don't rely on sunscreens to protect you

Sunscreens are creams that prevent the ultraviolet part of the sun's light spectrum from penetrating the skin, and should therefore prevent the damage that leads to cancer. Logically, their regular use by people constantly in the sun, whether on holiday or at work, should lead to a fall in cancer cases. That is certainly the intention of their makers, and the public have taken to these products in their millions. No one goes on sunshine holidays today without buying a sunscreen, and everyone knows that the higher the number on the tube, the longer they can stay in the sun.

The factor system depends on straight multiplication of the time you can spend in the sun without burning. If you can normally lie in the sun for only three minutes or so before you start to burn, then a Factor 5 cream should allow you 15 minutes and a Factor 15 cream lets you cook gently for three-quarters of an hour. Theoretically, on this scale, a total sunblock should allow you to bake for a whole day, but you would sweat away the remnants of your cream long before that time.

Soon after the introduction of sunscreens, dermatologists began to worry about their consequences. Had the popularity of sunblocks increased, rather than protected against, the risks of skin cancers? They reasoned that if people used sunscreens to stay longer in the sun than they otherwise would have done, and the creams were not as protective as they were claimed to be, the risk of cancer might rise rather than fall.

It is very difficult to prove an effect of a preparation against cancer, especially as skin cancers may take years to develop after the initial damage from the sun. They may remain unnoticed for 20 years or more before they grow enough to become obvious. We have not yet been using sunscreens for long enough to know for sure whether they have protected against skin cancers or have, by allowing people to stay longer in the sun, even increased their numbers.

Professor Michael E. Bigby of Harvard University addressed this in June 2004, in a commentary in *Archives of Dermatology*, an American Medical Association publication (Bigby, 2004). He had searched through every article published from 1966 to 2003 that reported on the use of sunscreens and melanoma in humans. He concluded that they showed no relationship between melanoma and sunscreen use. This was reassuring in one sense, in that sunscreens did not cause people to over-expose themselves to sun and therefore increase their risk of melanoma. But it was disappointing in another sense, in that sunscreens seem not to have prevented or lowered the risk of melanoma.

Professor Bigby stated that it was now time to dispense with the sunscreen and melanoma controversy. From his scrutiny of the data, there was no credible evidence that sunscreen use increases the risk of melanoma. He added 'we should continue to advocate that our patients avoid sun exposure to prevent skin cancer, including melanoma. Measures should include avoiding midday sun, wearing protective clothing, and the proper use of sunscreens. At the same time they should be cautioned not to use sunscreens to increase the amount of time they spend in the sun.'

The opposition to Professor Bigby's advice

Not everyone agrees with Professor Bigby's advice, and it would be remiss of me not to put forward a cogent view that has been expressed by a much respected British medical journalist and colleague of mine, Oliver Gillie. He is at odds with the orthodox view on the sun and skin cancer debate to such an extent that he has mounted what can only be described as a crusade against the advice to avoid the sun. His views are in broad agreement with those of Dr Kendrick that have been quoted earlier in this chapter, and I have included them here for the sake of completeness. Oliver has presented them in a series of bulleted points, which I reproduce below, word for word:

- The sun avoidance policy promoted each summer by government and by Cancer Research UK (CRUK) increases Vitamin D deficiency, putting the public at increased risk of serious chronic disease, including cancer.
- Insufficient Vitamin D is associated with, and is almost certainly a contributory cause of, several types of cancer, including cancer of the breast, prostate and bowel, as well as melanoma, the most serious form of skin cancer. Evidence suggests that Vitamin D deficiency is also a contributory cause of multiple sclerosis, hypertension and diabetes as well as causing the classic bone diseases of rickets, osteoporosis and osteomalacia.
- In the UK, most people get about 90 per cent of their Vitamin D from the sun. About 50 per cent of the UK population has insufficient levels of Vitamin D in the body.
- Evidence shows that people who spend more time in the sun are less likely to get melanoma (and probably other cancers) than people who avoid the sun. Those who are repeatedly burnt by the sun have a small increased risk of melanoma.
- CRUK's SunSmart policy advises people to avoid the sun from 11 a.m. to 3 p.m., to put on sunscreen half an hour before going out in the sun, and to cover up with clothes and a hat. This policy, if taken seriously, is likely to cause Vitamin D deficiency and consequent chronic disease in the long run. CRUK's SunSmart policy appears to be based on an Australian programme with the same name and is totally unsuited to the UK climate.
- CRUK has advised that people in the UK obtain enough Vitamin D from casual exposure of the hands and face. However, there is no scientific basis for this opinion and it is no longer supported by the UK National Radiological Protection Board.
- The government has spent more than a million pounds on advising the public to avoid the sun. The Chief Medical Officer's sixth tip for healthy living advises 'cover up, keep in the shade, never burn and use Factor 15 plus sunscreen'. This advice, like that of CRUK, is likely to cause Vitamin D deficiency and consequent chronic disease.

- More appropriate up-to-date advice for people in the UK is: sunbathe wearing as few clothes as possible whenever you get an opportunity, but take care not to bake or burn. The length of time it is advisable to stay in the sun will vary with skin type, previous exposure, time of day, time of year, clearness of sky, and latitude. Five to ten minutes' exposure every day all year round will provide a large amount of Vitamin D and maximum production of Vitamin D will be obtained after half an hour.
- The cost of treating diabetes is about £1.3 billion in the UK. The cost of treating hip fractures (mostly in old people suffering from osteoporosis) is £1.7 billion. Greater exposure to sunlight, which is free, could substantially reduce these costs and the even greater costs associated with cancer treatment.

Oliver puts forward a persuasive case, and I must say I see few flaws in it. There are more details at the website: <http://www.health researchforum.org.uk>.

I write a weekly medical column for various newspapers in Britain. Obviously I am concerned to present to my readers an unbiased judgement on medical subjects based on the most up-to-date respected scientific opinion of the time. When I decided to do this for sun exposure and skin cancer, it became clear that there were two factions with views that were difficult to reconcile. On the side of restriction of sun exposure to the minimum are the big guns of cancer and dermatology, such as Professor Bigby, CRUK, and the UK Chief Medical Officer of Health, along with most dermatologists. On the other side are the 'mavericks' such as Dr Kendrick and Oliver Gillie who want people to enjoy more sunshine and avoid other illnesses, and argue that more exposure to the sun will even prevent some melanomas. 'Mavericks' have a long and honourable history in British medicine: they have from time to time been proved right in the long run. Perhaps the Gillie/Kendrick view will prevail in the end.

I'm not sure, from his publications, exactly where Professor Weinstock stands on the issue – perhaps where I do, not quite on the fence. Here is what I wrote for my medical column. It is what I would say to a patient of mine who asked advice about prevention of skin cancer. I hope that it is a fair résumé of this chapter, and that the advice I give will not put anyone at any higher risk of cancer, of the skin or of an internal organ, than he or she was when they entered my consulting room.

A *summary of skin exposure to the sun and cancer*

We have all heard that numbers of cases of skin cancer have been increasing, and that the rise is largely, if not entirely, due to our desire to spend much more time in the sun. The message has been repeated so often that it is getting boring – and there's no indication that many people are actually heeding it. There's no sign that holidays in the Mediterranean, the Caribbean, the Far East and Australia are less popular than they were because they are places where there is too much sunshine.

Maybe the messages are wrong. They are just so severe that people prefer not to believe them. And there is another side to the sun. We all feel pleasure at the warmth of the sun on our skin. It does us good. People in sunny countries have lower rates of cancers of the breast, bowel, ovary and prostate and of non-Hodgkin's lymphoma (a cancer of the lymphatic system) than people in Britain. Sun on our skin makes Vitamin D, that's needed to make bones strong. It may also directly prevent development of internal cancers.

So there's an argument that although we may stimulate skin cancer if we sunbathe, it is more than offset by the protection it gives against other cancers and illnesses such as multiple sclerosis, rheumatoid arthritis, Type 1 diabetes and Crohn's disease, all of which seem to be relatively rare in sunny climates.

It is an impressive argument – until you hear the figures for the increase in skin cancers in Britain. Cases of melanoma, the most malignant type of skin cancer, have risen by *2,000 per cent* in the last 60 years. People born in 1935 could have expected a one in fifteen hundred chance of developing the disease in their lifetime. For people born in 2000 that chance is now 1 in 74 and, if we don't change our habits, it may even be as high as 1 in 7.

These figures are from Professor Martin Weinstock, a world expert in skin cancers. He wants to change the usual messages about skin cancer to make them more acceptable.

The first was 'avoid the sun'. Professor Weinstock stresses that if you really need to avoid the sun (and not everyone does), then you should eat plenty of foods containing Vitamin D or take a Vitamin D supplement when you do so. That may help protect against illnesses that might occur if you are not getting the vitamin from sunshine.

Message two is 'tanning is unhealthy'. People whose forebears came from Africa, South Asia or the Mediterranean, with their natural tans, have much less chance of developing skin cancers than pale-skinned northern Europeans. In fact, they need to expose their skin to the sun. Darker skin makes less Vitamin D than paler skin, and living under cooler cloudier northern skies can leave browner people with Vitamin D deficiency. They, too, must eat healthily, and if necessary take a Vitamin D supplement.

But if you have pale skin that burns in the sun and only tans with difficulty, then a tan is unhealthy. In your case it is a sign of damage to the skin that can lead to a cancerous change. Professor Weinstock's message is 'the healthiest colour for your skin is the one you were born with'. He puts the 2,000 per cent rise in melanoma squarely on the 'pursuit of a tan by activities such as sunbathing and tanning lamps' by people with naturally pale skins. If you are pink or pale, by all means enjoy the sun on your skin, but do protect it with a sunscreen and a wide-brimmed hat, and a light shirt, don't sunbathe for too long, and don't let your skin become red and sore. The fairer you are, the more protection you need and the shorter should be your time in the sun.

That message applies equally to adults and children. If you are pink, don't try to go brown in the sun. The cancer process can start at any age, and not just in children. It just isn't worth risking it.

Dr Tom Smith, *Bradford Telegraph & Argus*, 11 October 2005

The following chapters describe the main types of skin cancer and how you can learn to recognize them early. The case histories in Chapter 1 were an introduction to them: now we are going into more detail.

4

Common non-cancerous skin lumps and lesions

Everyone has skin blemishes. We call them freckles, moles, birth-marks, warts, cysts or even just spots. Most of the time we don't bother about them: we probably don't even notice them. It's only when they start to change, in shape, size or colour, or when you or a relative reads a book like this, that you start to worry and make an appointment to see your GP.

Much more often than not, you are then reassured. The vast majority of skin 'lesions' seen by family doctors turn out to be benign, and unrelated to cancer. For the following study results I'm indebted to Dr Scott M. Strayer of the University of Virginia Health Service, in Charlottesville, USA, for his report on the diagnosis of skin cancers (Strayer, Reynolds and colleagues, 2003). He and his team studied 1,215 biopsies of skin lesions in men and women who had come to them because of a concern that they might have skin cancer. Although Dr Strayer and his colleagues practise in the USA, their patients are of a similar ethnic and racial mix to most areas of the UK, and their climate is temperate, rather than subtropical, so that their results probably closely reflect the British and northern European experience.

More than 80 per cent of the 1,215 biopsies were diagnosed as benign; they included:

- Naevi
- Seborrhoeic keratosis
- Dermatofibromas and histiocytomas
- Cysts
- Lipomas
- Skin tags

If your skin problem has been given one of these labels, you can be reassured. They do not turn into cancers. They are explained below, so that you can recognize for yourself the ways in which they differ from cancers.

Naevi

Everyone's skin has 'moles' or, to use the correct name, naevi. In our student dermatology classes we were taught that moles are small furry animals that burrow underground and are only malign towards lawns, and that attitude has stuck with me over the years. However, most people call brown patches on the skin 'moles', so I'll use the word here and hope that I don't offend my former teachers. Moles vary in colour from light brown to much darker, and in size from a small spot to a larger patch up to 4 or 5 centimetres across. The average adult has between 10 and 20 pigmented (brown or black) moles (see Figure 2).

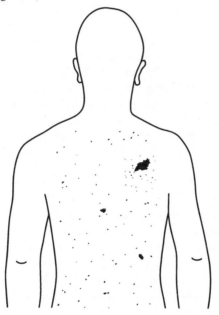

Figure 2 Pigmented naevi

The density of their colour depends on the numbers and activity of the melanocytes underneath them at the junction between the dermis and the epidermis. The higher the numbers and the more active they are in producing melanin, the blacker their colour. As we age, the melanocytes 'drop down' deeper into the dermis, to produce 'compound naevi', which may be the same colour as the rest of our skin, or brown, and may have hairs growing from them. Moles like this can appear for the first time in large numbers during puberty and in pregnancy. Their sudden 'eruption', especially as they are brown, tends to convince people that they may be cancerous.

They are not. When they appear like this, they are not malignant and do not become cancerous, but many people would like them removed, if only for cosmetic reasons, and they can be cut out surgically or by diathermy (cauterization – using heat). There is one proviso here. Babies born with extensive dark brown hairy naevi should have them removed and skin grafts placed over the resulting defect in the skin. These 'moles' do carry an increased risk of becoming malignant later.

Newborn babies may also have 'warty naevi' on their neck or face, or even in a line extending down an arm or leg. They look like the sort of warts that children 'catch' later, but such warts (see below, in the second paragraph on keratosis), are not the result of infections. They look more yellow than the usual wart, and microscope study shows that they contain sweat glands and hair follicles, none of which are in viral warts. They are best removed by a plastic surgeon, who will usually 'shave' them off.

Seborrhoeic keratosis

Sebum is an oily substance produced by sebaceous glands in the skin. Seborrhoea is over-production of the sebaceous glands, which most people would recognize in the spots of acne, when the sebaceous glands around the nose and cheeks swell and become blocked as the sebum solidifies. Acne subsides with time, leaving small pits in the skin that are the remains of the openings to the now redundant sebaceous glands.

The common word for keratosis is a wart. At some time in our childhood, most of us sprout warts on our fingers and feet. They are infections of the epidermis with wart viruses. They, too, subside with time, leaving no scar, as our immune systems deal with the infection, which is entirely within the superficial levels of the epidermis.

A seborrhoeic keratosis therefore is a wart that derives from the sebaceous glands. They arise not in childhood, but in older middle age, from our forties onwards, anywhere on our bodies (often across the back) in almost everyone. They start as a pale-yellow or brown pimple (the medical word is 'papule'), a small smooth lump raised from the surface of the skin, and they feel slightly greasy – this is their covering of sebum. From that stage they continue to grow, usually becoming darker or even black, and develop a flattened, dimpled surface, so that they become much more recognizable as a wart. People often feel that these 'warts' are 'stuck on' to the skin, and not growing outwards from it. They may be movable as if they are attached by a 'stalk' – this is classified as a 'pedunculated' keratosis.

We are not sure why so many people develop seborrhoeic warts as they grow older: there may be a viral involvement, but so far it has not been discovered. Some older men find that their backs have become covered with them, and they may become anxious that their spread means that they may be cancerous. However, they can be reassured: whatever causes these seborrhoeic warts, they never become malignant. They are removed because they are unsightly or because they catch on clothing, such as a bra strap or braces.

Extremely rarely, seborrhoeic warts appear in very large numbers in just a few weeks. This is called the 'Leser-Trélat sign', and is connected with the early development of a cancer of the bowel or other internal organs; so if this is happening to you, see your doctor immediately.

Seborrhoeic warts may be removed under a local anaesthetic either by curettage or freezing ('cryotherapy').

Dermatofibromas and histiocytomas

Dermatofibromas affect mainly the legs and arms, although they are sometimes found on other parts of the body. They occur more often in men than in women, perhaps because women's limbs are more likely to be uncovered by clothing than men's. They are small firm lumps ('nodules'), about the size and feel of a lentil, and are firmly lodged within the skin, rather than underneath it. They are thought to be a reaction to a previous injury, possibly an insect bite. Early on in their development they are softer in feel, and when removed and examined under the microscope they contain a mass of 'histiocytes' – large 'white' tissue cells whose purpose is to 'scavenge' any foreign material (such as insect saliva and cells) that may be present under the skin after a bite. At this stage, before fibrosis (scarring), they are called histiocytomas.

Some histiocytomas may contain masses of small blood vessels, so that they look very pink. If they are knocked, they may bleed into the skin, leaving a permanent brown mark where iron has been deposited. Specialists call this a 'sclerosing angioma'.

Dermatofibromas, histiocytomas and sclerosing angiomas never become malignant, and can be removed quite easily under local anaesthetic.

Cysts

Cysts are fluid-filled lumps. They are rare in the skin, but they can grow from a sweat gland or a hair follicle, the outlet of which has become blocked. Acne spots could be considered a form of cyst, but more common are cysts that form in the armpit from sweat glands, or the 'ganglions' that form on the tendons of the front of the wrist. Tendons run inside lubricated sheaths, and if adhesions (perhaps due to tiny traumas from repeated finger work) cause the tendon to stick to the sheath, the lubricating fluid can collect in the space between the tendon and its covering. The wrist is the most common place for this to happen.

Cysts are usually under, rather than in, the skin, so that you can move the surface skin freely over them: they are not embedded in the skin in the way that dermatofibromas are. If the fluid within them is clear, a pen-torch light will shine through them. They can be 'collapsed' by sucking out the fluid within them with a syringe and needle, or burst by hitting them with a heavy object (in the case of ganglions, the tradition was to use a family Bible!). Hitting with a hard object works best with a ganglion, but other types of cyst (such as a large sebaceous cyst) tend to grow again, and the best cure is to remove them surgically.

Cysts do not become cancerous.

Lipomas

You can look on a lipoma as a cyst full of fat, rather than fluid. Lipomas are smooth, usually soft, lumps that are also under the skin, in the fatty tissues below the dermis, so they can, like most cysts, be moved about easily between your finger and thumb. They may grow steadily over a long time, perhaps years, or remain at their original size. They are very common: many people who are a little overweight have several lipomas on their limbs and bodies. They don't become malignant, and are almost always easily removed under local anaesthetic.

Skin tags

Skin tags are those small lumps, rather like tiny warts, that women, especially those with brown eyes and hair, notice around the neck and in their armpits. They can grow elsewhere on the body. Although most skin tags remain the size of a mustard seed, they can sometimes grow to the size of a hazel nut. A few contain melanin and are really moles that have grown away from the skin surface.

It's common to mistake skin tags for a cluster of warts, but they are simply small collections of un-desquamated skin connected to the surface by a 'pedicle' or stalk. They are easily removed by nipping them off at the base of their stalk, or even by tying a surgical thread around them. Although it's natural to view the sudden appearance of skin tags as a possible sign of spreading cancer, skin tags never become malignant.

Other skin conditions

Molluscum contagiosum

Molluscum contagiosum mainly affects children. It is an infection with a 'pox' virus, related to chickenpox and cowpox, which produces small dome-shaped papules (pimples) with a central depression – a pimple with a dimple. When they arise in children they are easily recognized by the GP, and the family can be reassured that they will last for between 6 and 12 months, then disappear on their own, without treatment. It is more difficult to diagnose if a single molluscum contagiosum spot appears on an adult's face, as it then looks very like an early basal cell cancer (see Chapter 5). It may be diagnosed only after the lesion is removed surgically and examined under the microscope.

Keloid

Keloids appear after the skin has been wounded, as after an operation or a burn. It is a thickened, raised, firm mass of fibrous tissue that forms instead of the thin line of a normal healing scar, and its rapid growth can suggest to people that it might be cancerous, but it is not. It is the result of over-production of collagen in the wound space as a response to the injury, and has an underlying genetic cause.

Recognized early, it can be treated by applying a pressure dressing for the first few weeks until the healing process settles down. Steroid drugs can be injected into the keloid to reduce the amount of newly formed collagen. Keloids should not be removed surgically, as the new scar will only produce another keloid.

'Pre-malignant' lesions

Some 80 per cent of the skin lesions seen by Drs Strayer and Reynolds were in the benign categories listed above – which leaves 20 per cent that were malignant or in a category that is defined as pre-malignant. The latter is a group of skin conditions that, if left to develop without being removed or treated, has a high likelihood of becoming cancerous.

The two main pre-malignant conditions are actinic keratoses and lentigo maligna. They made up 7 per cent of the 1,215 skin lesions biopsied by Drs Strayer and Reynolds.

Actinic keratoses

Actinic, solar or senile keratoses (there are three names for the same lesions) form in skin that has been in the sun for long periods, usually many years. The paler your skin is, and the more intense the sunshine (in other words, the nearer the Equator you live), the shorter the time it takes for keratoses to appear. At first they are more easily felt than seen, as small areas of roughened skin, mainly on the face, the temples and forehead, a bald head, or the backs of the hands. They may grow a little larger, but it is more likely that more small keratoses appear with continuing sun exposure. They can turn into squamous cell cancers, but this is in fact quite rare, with perhaps less than 1 in 100 doing so, and then only after a long time.

Keratoses caused by sun exposure can usually be managed by your GP. If there are only one or two, then they can be cauterized, frozen or cut away, but there may be too many of them to do so with ease. An alternative is to apply a cream containing 5-fluorouracil (5-FU) twice daily after first washing the area with soap and water. The anti-cancer drug targets cells that are in 'mitosis' – in the act of dividing into two daughter cells in order to increase in number. As cancer cells are much more likely to be in mitosis than normal skin cells, they absorb the drug selectively, and die off. In effect, 5-FU is a 'golden bullet' killing off cancer cells while preserving most of the normal cells.

If you have been asked to use 5-FU you must understand that the skin becomes red and sore after a few days, but that you must continue to use it, and put up with the soreness for six weeks. Once the treatment has finished, you may need an antibiotic cream to deal with any infection, but you will be left without a scar, and with normal skin. Most people feel that the treatment is worthwhile, and of course it has the added bonus of preventing any cancer developing on the treated area of skin.

Lentigo maligna

Benign lentigo is a flat brown spot that appears in older people on skin that has been exposed to the sun. Examined under the microscope, it shows more than the usual numbers of melanocytes in the epidermal basal layer: this differentiates it from freckles, in which there is no increase in melanocyte numbers. It is classified as lentigo maligna when the spot is on the cheek, is more than 2 centimetres in diameter, and shows different shades of brown, blue or black on its surface. Lentigo is in fact a melanoma that has not yet spread to other areas, and has a high risk of becoming malignant, so it should be treated as a melanoma. The modern treatment of melanoma is described in Chapter 9.

Bowen's disease

This section on pre-malignant lesions would not be complete without a mention of Bowen's disease. Curiously, it does not feature in the paper by Drs Strayer and Reynolds, perhaps because none of the patients in their sample had it. However, my own experience of several practices in rural Scotland suggests that there are one or two patients with it in most practices. Angela's case described in Chapter 1 is typical.

Bowen's disease, or intra-epidermal carcinoma (it is also called carcinoma-in-situ of the skin), develops in people over 50 years old and looks just like a red patch of eczema or psoriasis. Because of that, it may well go undiagnosed for years before the patient and doctor realize that it is steadily enlarging, is constantly desquamating (shedding scaly pieces of skin), and yet does not itch or respond to the usual anti-eczema or anti-psoriasis treatments. A close look shows that it is flatter than most patches of psoriasis and does not weep like eczema. It is well demarcated from the surrounding skin with a very irregular edge, and often covers a large area – perhaps 5 to 10 centimetres across or occasionally more. Thankfully, although it can turn into an invasive squamous cell cancer, it very rarely does so. Nevertheless, it should be treated, either by surgery (often with a skin graft to cover the defect in the skin that is left) or by 5-FU used in the same way as for solar keratoses. Freezing or irradiating small areas are options best left to the specialist.

A year's experience as a GP in relation to skin cancer

In the experience of Drs Strayer and Reynolds, in each year a family doctor in a busy practice diagnoses six or seven basal cell cancers, one or two squamous cell cancers, and perhaps one malignant melanoma. Their experience is based on the east coast of the USA, at a latitude close to that of the northern Mediterranean, so they may be seeing more cases of melanoma than the average GP in the UK. In Scotland, despite the recent rises in melanoma cases here, I'm sure we see fewer melanomas than they do. My experience of basal and squamous cell cancers, however, is about the same as theirs.

Although they are much rarer than other skin cancer types, making sure that we don't miss a melanoma is exceptionally important for family doctors. Although they form only 1 per cent of skin malignancies, melanomas account for more than three-quarters of the deaths from them. More than 90 per cent of people with the diagnosis of squamous and basal cell cancers are still alive, well and free from recurrence after five years. The cure rate for recurrent malignant melanoma is under 50 per cent. However, every year this is improving. The following chapters, based on earlier diagnosis of skin cancers and on modern approaches to their cure, explain why this is happening.

5

Non-melanoma skin cancers – types and tests

In the previous chapter you read that 80 per cent of all people who come to their family doctors worried about a possible skin cancer receive the good news that their lesions are benign. A further 7 per cent have lesions, such as solar keratosis, lentigo maligna or Bowen's disease, that may become cancers, but can be treated before they do so.

That leaves 13 per cent who are given the bad news that they have skin cancer. In the studies presented by Drs Strayer and Reynolds, of these people 73 per cent had a basal cell cancer (BCC), 14 per cent had a squamous cell cancer (SCC) and 12 per cent had a malignant melanoma. In 1 per cent, the lesions were secondary deposits in the skin from internal malignant tumours. These US statistics are probably similar to those in the UK, with the proviso that their melanoma figures are probably higher than ours. We may not have to wait long, however, before we catch up with the USA. That may be the price we are about to pay for our huge increase in sunshine holidays.

Basal cell cancers – BCCs

BCC is now the most common of all cancers in the USA and Australia, and is on the way to becoming the most common form in the UK too. BCCs usually form on the face (see Figure 3), nearly always in people over the age of 50, but they *can* occur at any site and in younger adults. A typical BCC starts as a small, smooth lump that grows slowly over months and years to a round doughnut-shaped mound with a central depression. Within the 'doughnut' area there are small pearl-coloured areas, and over the rim are tiny red blood vessels. The central pit can become an ulcer with a crust over it: removing the crust reveals the pearly edge.

Unfortunately, in making an early diagnosis, not all BCCs are typical. Dermatologists divide BCCs into 'superficial', which remain on the surface of the skin; 'pigmented', which may be various shades of brown or blue-black, and could be mistaken for melanoma;

and 'infiltrating', in which a central ulcer 'bores into' the skin into the tissues beneath it. They can also be 'nodular', in which they remain as a single smooth lump in the skin; 'cystic', with a hollow centre; 'morphoeic', in which the skin thickens into a waxy ivory-coloured 'plaque' or disc; and keratotic, in which it is like a wart.

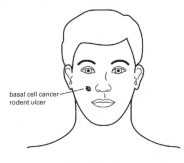

basal cell cancer
rodent ulcer

Figure 3 Basal cell cancer/rodent ulcers (BCCs)

The message from all this is that if you have a 'spot' on your skin that has arisen out of the blue, and it does not fade away naturally over a week or so, get your doctor to examine it. There is a high chance that it is one of the benign conditions described in the previous chapter, but you cannot ignore the possibility that it may be a BCC.

A common way for a BCC to be diagnosed is for a man to complain that he has a small crusty area on his cheek that bleeds when he shaves. He 'keeps taking the top off' with the razor blade, and it 'never seems to heal'. A woman may notice a similar spot when applying her make-up. She needs to take extra time over that area of skin, and it begins to annoy her. Both man and woman, in these circumstances, are surprised, even shocked, when told the diagnosis.

Happily for them and for everyone with a BCC, it is the least lethal of all skin cancers. BCCs do not spread distantly to other organs or areas of the body. However, they may, if left alone, erode deeper into the tissues below the skin, even into bone, leaving a large unsightly ulcer on the face that can become infected. So all skin lesions that are suspected of being an early BCC should be removed and the tissues examined under a microscope.

Microscope examination of a BCC will not only confirm the diagnosis by identifying the type of cell (the basal cell) that has become cancerous, it will also give a fair idea of the likely outcome – in medical terms, the prognosis. The pathologist will take into account the tumour size, the site from which it has been removed (face, forehead, scalp, a lip margin, an eyelid), the type of cell and its activity (what proportion of the cells are in an active phase of reproducing themselves), and whether the whole tumour has been removed at the operation (that is, decide on whether or not there is a clear margin of normal tissues all round the cancerous cells).

The prognosis will be more guarded if the person has had a previous BCC or if this is a repeat operation on a previous BCC that has not been cured. Your doctors will also be more circumspect about your prognosis if you have an immune problem (if you have had an organ transplant or have an illness that has lowered your immune system's ability to combat infection or cancer).

After taking all these features of your case into account, your doctors will then categorize you as low or high risk. Only then will the treatment choices be discussed with you. The treatments for BCC are discussed in Chapter 6.

Squamous cell cancers – SCCs

SCCs are the second most common skin cancers. They are usually related to sun exposure over long periods in people who tend to burn quickly, rather than tan, in the sun. It is especially common, therefore, in fair-skinned, blue-eyed people who react to the sun by going red, blistering, feeling sore, and who may freckle rather than go uniformly brown. Albinos, who cannot make protective melanin at all, have a very high risk of SCC. It is also a common complication of the chronic skin disease xeroderma pigmentosum, in which an inherited fault in the genes leads to an inability to repair completely skin burned by the sun. This leads to multiple areas of solar keratoses that eventually turn into SCC. People with xeroderma must stay out of direct sunlight and use high-factor sunscreens.

Not all SCCs are linked to the sun. Some arise on areas of skin that are normally covered by clothes, or on scars from old wounds or burns, including radiation or chemical burns. In the past, arsenic (unbelievably, used in ointments or creams in the nineteenth century) was a common cause of SCC development. SCCs may form in the edges of chronic ulcers, as in varicose or diabetic ulcers around the ankles.

People with immune system problems, such as those who have had a transplant or with lymphoma or leukaemia (cancers of the lymphatic system or the bone marrow) are also at higher than usual risk of having an SCC. If you are on long-term immunosuppression for one of these illnesses, you should avoid sunbathing, wear protective clothing, and use effective sunblocks.

SCCs start as a small lump, medically described as a 'nodule', which grows quite quickly, but not as fast as the kerato-acanthoma described in George's case in Chapter 1. They have a firm 'feel' and may form a thick crust of keratin that eventually erodes into a central ulcer. They may then grow outwards, like a miniature cauliflower, or remain flat on the skin, producing a shallow ulcer and no crust. In either case, an SCC will show no sign of healing, and people with an SCC tend to come to their doctor about it sooner than those with a BCC.

That is just as well, because SCCs have a bad habit of spreading to distant organs ('metastasis') and it is vital to cure them before they do so.

As with BCCs, the definitive diagnosis of an SCC is made from its examination under the microscope. A typical report from the pathologist will mention the pattern of the cells (do they look glandular or less structured?); the shape of the cells (spindle-shaped or round?); and their 'differentiation' (do they look like more mature cells, recognizable as squamous cells, or are they more primitive and immature?). The pathologist will also report on how far the tumour has invaded deeply into the skin, whether the whole tumour has been removed, and whether there is any extension of the tumour around the nerves, the blood vessels or lymphatic vessels nearby.

The pathologist will complete the report by estimating the risk of metastases. This depends on the site of the tumour, its size, rate of growth, the cause, the degree of differentiation (the less differenti-ated, the more likely it is to spread), and whether or not the person has lowered immunity.

In 2003, the *British Journal of Plastic Surgery* published guidelines for doctors for the management of patients with primary squamous cell cancer of the skin. The authors of these guidelines, Drs R. Motley, P. Kersey and C. Lawrence, wrote them on behalf of the British Association of Dermatologists, the British Association of Plastic Surgeons, and the Faculty of Clinical Oncology of the Royal College of Radiologists (Motley, Kersey and Lawrence, 2003). The next few paragraphs, outlining the way your doctor will assess the risk that your particular SCC may metastasize, are taken from those guidelines. They are certainly not meant to frighten you, but to give you an idea of what to ask about when you want to know your chances of complete cure. Keep strongly in your mind that we now have very high cure rates for SCC: they are currently well above 90 per cent and are still improving.

Assessing the risk of metastasis

Site of the tumour

SCCs that have started at sun-exposed sites, excluding the lip and ear, are least likely to spread. In order of increasing risk of spread, the next sites are the lip, then the ear, and tumours in non-sun-exposed sites such as the groin, lower back, and sole. Most likely to send off secondary cancers are SCCs in old areas of burns, radiation injury, chronic ulcers and SCCs that have arisen from a patch of Bowen's disease.

Size of the tumour

Tumours more than 2 centimetres in diameter have a 15 per cent chance of recurring on the same site after treatment, and a 30 per cent risk of metastasizing. The corresponding figures for smaller SCCs are 7 per cent and 9 per cent, so that the larger SCCs have twice the chance of spreading again locally, and three times the chance of spreading distantly to other organs than smaller SCCs. These numbers are a big incentive not to delay in seeking your doctor's advice about any doubtful skin lump or ulcer.

Differentiation

The microscopic appearance of the SCC matters. Poorly differenti-ated tumours (in which all the cells look 'primitive' and immature, and are rapidly dividing) have more than twice the local recurrence rate and three times the metastatic rate of well-differentiated tumours (in which the cells look much more like normal squamous cells and many fewer are undergoing cell division).

Tumours that look, under the microscope, as if they are spreading alongside nerve fibres are more likely to recur and to metastasize, but oddly that does not seem to be proven for tumours that seem to be spreading into blood or lymph vessels. Why this is so has not yet been discovered.

Immune suppression

If you are on immune suppressant drugs after a transplant or for other reasons, or if you have an illness that causes immune suppression, then your SCC is more likely to spread. A normal immune response is important, it seems, in preventing local or distant extension of a skin cancer of any type.

Previous and present treatment

The risk of spread to adjacent tissues depends to some extent on how your SCC has been, or is being, treated. If you have had an SCC before, and it has returned, then the risk of metastasis is higher. The recurrence rate is much less if your consultant uses Mohs' micrographic surgery. This will be explained in the treatment section for SCC in Chapter 6.

6

Treating non-melanoma skin cancers – (1) Basal cell cancers (BCCs)

The main aim in treating basal cell cancers (BCCs) is to get rid of all the cancer tissue. If any of it is left, it can continue to grow into the tissues beneath and around it. It is extremely unlikely to metastasize to other sites in the body, so that if it can be completely removed it is cured. Almost the same can be said for early squamous cell cancers (SCCs), which tend to spread elsewhere only when the primary tumour is in a later stage, so that only a very small proportion of people with SCCs eventually die from its spread.

On the basis that BCCs are now by far the most common type of skin cancer, this chapter will deal with their treatment. Chapter 7 covers SCCs – some of the treatments of which are common to those of BCCs.

(Malignant melanoma has different investigation and treatment priorities, and needs two chapters to itself: Chapters 8 and 9.)

The gold standard treatment for BCCs is surgery, preferably using a system called Mohs' micrographic surgery, in which the surgeon uses a microscope and chemical agents to define the margins and depth of the tumour, in order to be assured that all of it is removed at the first operation. Professor F. E. Mohs had a long and active career in skin cancer, publishing his first paper in 1941 on the surgical technique that is named after him. By 1976, he was still writing about the ways in which his method could be updated (Mohs, 1941 and 1976).

Mohs' micrographic surgery

Mohs' micrographic surgery for a first BCC produces an overall five-year cure rate of 99 per cent, and for recurrent BCCs the corresponding figure is 95 per cent (Rowe and colleagues, 1989). These are far higher success rates than for any other medical or surgical treatment method for skin cancers, so why is it not used by everyone, in every case? One excuse is that surgeons using the method need special expertise and training: it is much more expensive than the usual outpatient treatments for BCC.

Many hospitals therefore restrict Mohs' surgery to those whose BCCs put them in a high-risk category. In other words, they have BCCs on their eyelids, ears, lips, nose or the fold between the nose and cheek. Their BCCs are invasive deep into the surrounding skin and are more than 2 centimetres in diameter. Under the microscope, they show spread along the line of nerves. BCCs that have recurred at the site of a previous operation must also be treated using the Mohs' method.

Although these high-risk features seem to form a long list, they still exclude most BCCs, which carry a much lower risk and can be adequately treated with other less exacting methods. These include, apart from more routine surgery, curettage, cautery, electrodesiccation, cryosurgery, laser therapy and radiotherapy. There is also photodynamic therapy and creams such as 5-FU that are specific for skin tumours. BCCs have been injected with interferon (see p. 56), and the very rare people whose BCCs have metastasized have been given chemotherapy. The next few pages describe these other methods and their success rates.

Other surgery

Surgery is the treatment of choice for most BCCs. It is not enough just to remove the BCC: a wide margin of surrounding healthy skin has to be taken as well, to ensure that all of the lesion (including the microscopic areas of spread not visible to the eye, which can't be felt, even by a surgeon's sensitive fingers), is removed. For a well-defined BCC under 2 centimetres in diameter, this margin is around 4 millimetres, and will remove the whole tumour in 95 per cent of cases. The bigger the BCC or the closer it is to high-risk areas, the wider the margin must be. Tumours that have penetrated into the tissues under the dermis, or that are in particularly dangerous areas, such as the eyelids, ears, lips and nose described above for Mohs' surgery, are given a wider margin – of 6 millimetres or more. If you have had treatment for a BCC before, and it has recurred, the margin may have to be as wide as 10 millimetres. These wider margins should make sure that any microscopic spread into the surrounding tissues, which the surgeon will not be able to see directly, is removed along with the main tumour.

Obviously, taking a margin of normal skin as well as the tumour may mean that a skin graft has to be applied to fill in the defect that is left. Therefore such operations are best performed by highly skilled plastic surgeons who are very experienced in this area. It is not just a matter of your family doctor, or even a general surgeon or dermatologist, performing such operations alongside their other daily tasks. This is especially so for the face, where scarring can be extremely distressing.

If you are in the high-risk category you should be treated by a multiprofessional oncology team, involving a dermatologist, pathologist, a surgeon appropriately trained in plastic or maxillo-facial surgery, a clinical oncologist and a clinical nurse with special training in skin cancer. Before you undergo surgery you should be given full information about the diagnosis, the type and extent of your treatment, your prognosis, and your follow-up support. You should be given the opportunity to sign a consent form to the treatment once you have understood all its ramifications.

Curettage, cautery and cryotherapy

Not everyone wants, or is suitable for, surgery, and many dermatologists prefer to use other techniques for those with BCCs that are relatively small, are not on crucial sites, and are low risk. The most common approaches for these BCCs are curettage (scraping out the centre with a 'spoon'), cautery (burning off the cancer), and cryotherapy (freezing it).

The choice of which of these you will be offered depends mainly on the experience of the dermatologist and his or her preferences. They are usually performed under local anaesthetic, although those who are anxious and those with larger BCCs may be offered a general anaesthetic. In low-risk sites and for small BCCs, five-year cure rates (without recurrence in that time) are around 95 per cent. Tumour size is important here: as the diameter rises above 1 centimetre, recurrence rates rise steeply. Also important is that the treatment is the first for that particular BCC. If a BCC recurs, a second use of these treatments brings only a 60 per cent rate of cure. Surgery is a much better option in such cases.

There are several types of cryotherapy, using open or closed sprays, and giving the tumour single, double or even three exposures to a freeze-thaw cycle. Most studies of cryotherapy specifically exclude its use on high-risk BCCs, especially on eyelids, ears and nose. There are reports that it has benefits on eyelids, but one drawback is that it can cause a hole in the eyelid that eventually needs plastic surgery to repair it.

My own strong opinion from reading the literature and from my experience in patients over the years is that if you have the option of surgery for a BCC, you should take it. However, this is a personal opinion, and if you are about to have a BCC treated, your dermatologist has every right to help you towards another decision.

Radiotherapy

Today in the UK many skin cancer patients are looked after by a team consisting of a dermatologist, a clinical oncologist and a plastic surgeon. Your oncologist may offer radiotherapy for your BCC. Radiotherapy is extremely useful, but you can be sure that if that is what is offered to you, there has been a very careful selection process before the decision was reached.

In a series of 93 people whose BCCs were irradiated, the two-year cure rate was 96 per cent (Hall and colleagues, 1986), and a review of many studies undertaken since 1945 reports a five-year cure rate of 90 per cent, although it must be admitted that its authors concluded that Mohs' surgery was their preference (Rowe and colleagues, 1989).

Radiotherapy can be used in many sites, but it is less suitable for larger BCCs because they are resistant to it and they require radiation doses that may burn and damage the normal tissues surrounding the BCC. It is also not used for younger adults because it may induce in later years changes in the skin such as atrophy (thinning and ageing) and telangiectasia (the appearance of small red blood vessels on the skin surface, which do not look attractive). The treatment also requires several visits to the cancer centre, rather than the single treatment of the other approaches. Scarring of the eyelid may also lead to constant weeping or an inward-turning lid, both of which are distressing.

Radiotherapy must therefore be chosen with care, and must be used only by a specialist with considerable knowledge of, and experience in, its use.

Topical therapy

Medically, 'topical' means a treatment applied to a surface, such as the skin, and is not used here in the sense of today's news or fashion! The 5-FU, or 5-fluorouracil, cream mentioned in Chapter 1 for treatment of solar keratoses has been used to treat BCCs, but has met with mixed success. The current consensus is that it can't be expected to cure BCCs, except for very small, early lesions, and the irritation it causes as the cancer cells die off would be very uncomfortable on BCCs on the face. Its use is probably best confined to multiple small and superficial BCCs on the body and legs.

Interferon-alpha

Interferon-alpha is a 'cytokine', part of the body's natural immune system that helps to control the body's responses to 'foreign' proteins, such as from a bacterium or virus, or from an allergen such as pollen, or the new proteins that are found in cancer cells. In the laboratory it has blocked the growth of cancer cells, so it was tried out in the treatment of BCCs. In the first study of direct injections of interferon-alpha into BCCs, all eight subjects were cured (Greenway and colleagues, 1986). Sadly, subsequent studies haven't confirmed such a high cure rate. In the first of these studies, in 172 cases of BCC, there was an immediate failure rate of 14 per cent and a recurrence rate within a year of another 19 per cent (Cornell and colleagues, 1990).

The mechanism by which interferon-alpha 'switches off' cancer cell activity is now well known: it stops the production in the tumour of another cytokine called interleukin-10, an action that stops the tumour cells multiplying and effectively tells them to 'commit suicide'. This is great in theory, but in practice it has too high a failure rate, and is very expensive and time-consuming. A considerable disadvantage is that it gives people the feeling that they have the 'flu, with headaches, fever, muscle pains and cold symptoms, probably because the body thinks it is mounting an immune challenge against a viral invader.

Interferon-alpha is therefore never going to be the preferred treatment for routine BCC. It is finding a use, however, in a low dose alongside other chemotherapy, for mycosis fungoides, in which it reduces the numbers of circulating cancer cells and leads to improvement in the skin.

Imiquimod

Although interferon-alpha has turned out to be disappointing, its successors are queuing up to replace it. The most successful one to date is imiquimod. It belongs to the class of 'immune response modifiers' and, when applied to BCCs, it induces the cancer cells to 'commit suicide', a process called apoptosis, which is explained later, in the chapter on malignant melanoma. The trials to date have been very encouraging, with very high response rates in superficial BCCs, and slightly less complete responses in deeper, nodular, tumours.

Imiquimod is spread on the lesion five times a week for a period of between 6 and 12 weeks. Unfortunately, it often causes itch, tenderness and burning where it is applied to the skin. The shorter the time interval between applications, the better is the response, but the greater are the side effects and the less patients can tolerate it, so the five-times weekly system is a fair compromise that most people can endure. So far, because of the skin's reaction to it, imiquimod has mainly been used for BCCs on the body, rather than the face, but these are early days for the treatment, and it will surely be modified to make it more tolerable. It is only the first of many more drugs in research that should revolutionize the treatment of BCCs.

Retinoids

Retinoids are derived from Vitamin A, which is a vital element for healthy skin. Its action in normal skin is to promote the peeling of the outer keratin layer at the correct rate. Because of that, Vitamin A derivatives have been used with some success in diseases in which the skin thickens, such as psoriasis. Of course, you can have too much of a good thing, even when it is a vitamin. Here is what Antarctic explorer Sir Douglas Mawson wrote about his experience of too much Vitamin A in 1913. His provisions had vanished down a crevasse (along with a companion) and he was left to eat his huskies in order to survive. He should not have eaten the liver, however, because it stores millions of units of Vitamin A, many times more than the upper tolerable level for humans:

> The sight of my feet gave me quite a shock, for the thickened skin of the soles had separated in each case as a complete layer. I did what appeared to be the best thing under the circumstances: smeared the new skin with lanoline and with bandages bound the skin soles back into place (Shearman, 1978).

Retinoids will probably not be used routinely for BCC treatment, but there may be a place for them in people with multiple solar keratoses that are at high risk of becoming BCCs. Kidney transplant patients, with their reduced immunity as a result of anti-rejection drugs, are possible candidates for their use. Tazarotene, a retinoid developed for psoriasis, has been shown to reduce BCCs after being applied to them daily for many months (Peris and colleagues, 1999). A one-year study of the retinoid called acitretin in kidney transplant patients produced a fall in numbers of solar keratoses and no new skin cancers (De Sevaux and colleagues, 2003). However, side effects, mainly consisting of a dry mouth and eyes, limited their use and tolerance.

Anti-inflammatories (COX-2 inhibitors, or coxibs)

COX-2 specific inhibitors are promising agents in the battle against cutaneous neoplasia (skin cancer). Further double-blinded, randomized, placebo-controlled trials in humans are warranted to define the role of celecoxib and other COX-2 inhibitors in the prevention and treatment of non-melanoma skin cancers.

Drs Arun Chakrabarty and John K. Geisse wrote the above for *Clinics in Dermatology* in 2004. What a difference a year makes. I am writing in 2005, after celecoxib was withdrawn from the market because of doubts about its safety and claims that it caused fatal heart attacks. Yet the sentiment is correct. COX-2 inhibitors are anti-inflammatory drugs that act on an enzyme system in the body called cyclo-oxygenase 2, hence their name. There are plenty of studies to show that in cancer cells (in the bowel and breast as well as the skin) COX-2 is highly active, and that if it is blocked, the cancer cell shuts down its ability to replicate and dies off.

There are therefore many studies of COX-2 inhibitors in various cancers, including BCCs and SCCs. Animal studies have shown that celecoxib, the first one to be produced and the first to be abandoned, did prevent the development of skin cancers. Whether they will ever be translated into full human studies remains to be seen.

Diets and 'health' supplements

It is impossible today to write a book on any illness without having to mention dietary supplements and herbal medicines. I must admit here that I am profoundly sceptical that they may make a difference to our susceptibility to cancer, but I decided to review the literature anyway and present what I have found in a hopefully unbiased way. Here it is.

The buzz-word among the health conscious is 'antioxidant'. Antioxidants have gained a reputation for preventing cancer, heart disease and dementia, along with other major illnesses. Sadly, when put to the test of scientific controlled trials, they rarely meet their expectations. The trials I report here are small, and few have placebo-treated controls: those that do have had doubtful results.

Let us start with beta-carotene. In a large randomized controlled study, beta-carotene was no better than placebo in preventing non-melanoma skin cancers. Vitamin C and Vitamin E come next. When taken together they allowed skin to tolerate the sun for longer before it became red (the technical term is that they increased the minimal erythema dose – erythema meaning reddening). Yet another study reported a significant reduction in ultraviolet light-induced erythema when the subjects were taking a combination of Vitamin C, Vitamin E and melatonin. Melatonin is another currently popular supplement more usually connected with helping people who work difficult hours, or who are jet-lagged, to sleep.

Another proposal is that eating a lot of fat can shorten the time from exposure to ultraviolet light to the start of a skin cancer. In an impressive and painstaking study, Dr H. S. Black reported that those people assigned to low-fat foods developed only one-fifth of the solar keratoses in the following 8 to 12 months compared with their high-fat-eating control subjects. It seems that if you are prone to developing skin cancer (see the high-risk groups and the case histories), a low-fat diet may help in preventing them.

Drink tea, too, is another message of the dietary researchers. Black and green tea from India and China contain substances called polyphenols that protect the skin against light-induced cancers. Admittedly this statement comes from animal research, and there is not yet proof that they are protective in humans. There are similar claims for 'procyanins' made from grape seeds. But before we all change to drinking tea and munching the seeds in our grapes, it may be better to wait for human trial results. They may be a long time coming, and most people would prefer their grapes made into wine, which doesn't include the seeds!

7

Treating non-melanoma skin cancers – (2) Squamous cell cancers (SCCs)

Squamous cell cancers (SCCs) have much in common with BCCs. They arise in solar keratoses, they are linked to sun exposure, and they are more common in fair-skinned than in darker-skinned people. They are also more common in people with suppressed or depressed immunity. Some have been linked (as is cervical cancer) with human papilloma virus infection (Harwood and colleagues, 1999). The main way in which they differ from BCCs is that they tend to spread (metastasize) to other parts of the body, and when they do so they are extremely difficult to cure. If caught early, before they spread, they have very high cure rates.

SCCs start as a firm nodule in the skin, which looks like a wart (keratinized SCC), or as a crusted tumour that forms an ulcer, or as a 'sore', an ulcer with no lump in the skin, which does not heal.

The diagnosis of SCC is made from the microscope, and it is graded according to the appearance of the cells, their level of activity (judged on the numbers of dividing – or multiplying – cells to be seen on the slide, and on any 'invasion' of the cells into surrounding tissues, including around nerves, blood vessels or lymph glands. This is described in much more detail in Chapter 5.

The main aim of treatment of SCCs is to remove them completely before they can metastasize, and to avoid causing a metastasis (called 'in transit' metastases) while this is being done. The aim is also to remove any secondary spread that has occurred near the tumour. More difficult to do, and sometimes impossible, is to identify and remove metastases that have 'seeded' elsewhere, in the lungs for example.

If you are facing SCC surgery, don't let this worry you: most SCCs carry a very low risk of spread, and today's cure rates are well above 90 per cent.

Surgery

The first choice and the one with the best results for SCCs, as with BCCs (see Chapter 6), is surgical removal. Because even small SCCs can 'send' tiny metastases into the tissues around them, the surgery has to be extensive, and the area of normal skin that has to be removed around what seems to be a small lump or ulcer can be an unpleasant surprise, even a shock, to someone expecting just a lump removal. The larger the tumour is, the further is its microscopic spread, and the wider is the margin of healthy skin that must be removed.

As with BCCs (see Chapter 6), many surgeons use Mohs' micrographic surgery to identify the tumour margins, but with SCC there is the added difficulty that there may be microscopic metastatic spread, which the method will not detect. Surgeons using the technique in SCC, therefore, will usually take a wider area away than with BCC. The technique tends to be used more in high-risk SCC cases, where wider removal of tissues around the tumour is difficult without causing difficulties for the person afterwards. Eyelids, the angle of the nose and ears are good examples. Whatever type of surgery is used, it is vital that enough tissue is removed to guarantee, as far as the surgeon can, that the whole cancer has been eradicated.

Curettage and cautery

Many groups have reported excellent results using curettage and cautery (see Chapter 6 for an explanation) in slow-growing SCCs under 1 centimetre in diameter with a mature rather than an undifferentiated microscopic appearance. The surgeons limit this treatment to these forms of SCC with the proviso that they are on skin areas that have been exposed to the sun, such as the forearms and the backs of the hands (see Figure 4). It is not used as a sole treatment in high-risk tumours or for recurrences.

Some surgeons use curettage first, because they can 'feel' from its soft consistency the extent of the tumour tissue, and can therefore estimate its extent. They curette the tumour, then apply cautery or 'electrodesiccation', in which an electric current is used to dry out the wound. This curettage-cautery process is repeated at least once, and often twice. After 'debulking' the tumour in this way, the surgeons can then use Mohs' micrographic surgery to complete the job. If it is appropriate, they can follow up the debulking with cryosurgery or radiotherapy, rather than surgery.

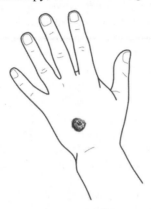

Figure 4 Squamous cell cancer

Cryosurgery

Some dermatologists offer cryotherapy (freezing with liquid nitrogen) for small SCCs. It can offer good results in experienced hands, but it is essential to have a pathology report first to confirm the diagnosis and that the tumour is not an aggressive one. The popularity of cryosurgery varies in different countries and between departments in hospitals in the same country or even region. My region is not enthusiastic about using it in anything but the earliest and least risky SCCs, and it is confined to departments where the staff are very well trained and experienced in its use.

Radiotherapy

Radiation therapy does work in SCCs: it gives comparable results to surgery, and in some cases will give a better appearance afterwards. It may be the choice for a tumour on a lip, or the inside surface of the nostril, and the ear, and is used for very advanced SCCs where the risk of surgery is high.

Lymph node dissection

There is ongoing debate about whether, for larger SCCs (more than 6 millimetres deep on the lip or more than 8 millimetres deep in other skin areas), the surgeon should also dissect out the nearest lymph nodes, to remove any microscopic metastasis that might be there. As a family doctor I'm not qualified to give an opinion on this, but Drs R. Motley, P. Kersey and C. Lawrence, of Cardiff, Plymouth and Newcastle upon Tyne, have given their opinion on behalf of the British Association of Dermatologists, the British Association of Plastic Surgeons and the Faculty of Clinical Oncology of the Royal College of Radiologists. I quote from their guidelines for the treatment of SCC: 'Elective lymph node dissection is not routinely practised and there is no compelling evidence of benefit over morbidity.'

I am glad of that, because from the family doctor's viewpoint it greatly increases the patient's discomfort, lengthens the healing time, and leaves a more unsightly scar, for no apparent advantage.

Follow-up

Simply treating the cancer is only the start. If you have SCC, your long-term survival depends first on whether or not you came to the doctor before the tumour spread to other areas of your body. It is highly likely that you did this, because the vast majority of people with SCCs are cured.

The second reason influencing your long-term survival is that the treatment has been appropriate: surgery for the high-risk SCCs and perhaps curettage and cryotherapy (possibly plus surgery) for less malign tumours.

The third is follow-up. Some 95 per cent of recurrences and of distant metastases are detected within five years of the initial operation. If you are alert to them and report them quickly, then you have every prospect of a further cure. So you should be on the hospital follow-up list for at least five years, and you should know how to examine your skin for any changes that might be suspicious. The cases of Margaret and William, in Chapter 1, although they are about melanoma, are an example to follow. Once you have had an SCC, you have a raised risk of a second. Don't be afraid of it, but be vigilant. When you know what you are looking for, and you become familiar with the details of your skin, you will notice something new in the same way that astronomers can pick out a comet or a supernova – just because it looks different from usual.

8

Diagnosing malignant melanoma

Malignant melanoma (MM) deserves a chapter to itself: it is the most complex of the skin cancers, and needs a different approach to diagnosis and treatment from BCCs and SCCs.

Here is Professor John F. Thompson of the University of Sydney melanoma unit, writing in the *Lancet* in 2005 (Thompson and colleagues, 2005):

> Melanoma has become a major public health problem in many countries. Since the mid 1960s melanoma incidence has risen by 3 to 8 per cent per year in most people of European background, with the greatest incidence in elderly men. Despite this increase the survival rate has improved substantially. Roughly 60 per cent of those diagnosed with melanoma in the 1960s died of the disease, compared with just 11 per cent more recently, an improvement attributed mainly to early detection.

The increase of 3 to 8 per cent per year does not sound much, but compounded over more than 40 years it is approaching 500 per cent, a figure not far from the 2,000 per cent since the 1930s mentioned earlier.

There is good news on melanoma: Professor Thompson reports that 85 per cent of people survive for at least five years after being diagnosed as having malignant melanoma. This is a big improvement on the 20 per cent of a generation ago, but Professor Thompson still isn't satisfied. He writes that in young adults melanoma still 'causes disproportionate mortality, so that an average of 18.6 years of potential life are lost for each melanoma death in the United States'.

Happily, greater public awareness of the causes of skin cancer, how to prevent it, and of the early signs of it, are combining, along with newer forms of treatment, to reduce the risks further. This chapter is about the causes, types, diagnosis and investigation of melanoma, and how there is much more knowledge today of all of these different aspects of the disease, including new approaches to defeating it.

Table 1 Risk factors for melanoma

	Relative risk (RR)
Genetic	
More than 3 close relatives affected (parent, sibling)	35–70
Weakly positive family history (1 relative affected)	3
Naevi (moles)	
Multiple (more than 100) benign naevi	11
Multiple compound or atypical naevi	11
Previous skin cancer	
Previous melanoma	8.5
Previous non-melanoma skin cancer	2.9
Immunosuppression	
Transplant recipients	3
AIDS patients	1.5
Skin sensitivity	
Skin burns without tanning	1.7
Freckles	2.5
Blue eyes	1.6
Red hair	2.4
UV exposure	
History of blistering sunburn	2.5

Source: Thompson and colleagues, 2005, p. 688.

First of all, Professor Thompson is as far from Oliver Gillie and Dr Kendrick as he can be about its cause. He is in no doubt that severe repeated episodes of sunburn in children correlates most closely with the risk of melanoma. Even if you are one of the unfortunate people born with a genetic mutation that predisposes you to melanoma (it is in a gene called CDKN2A), you are far more likely to develop one if you live nearer the Equator than if you live at a relatively high latitude, in a temperate zone such as northern Europe, Canada or the south island of New Zealand. Professor

Thompson lists the following as melanoma risk factors (see Table 1), and places beside them their relative risk (RR). An RR number of 11, for example, means that if you possess that factor, you increase your risk of developing malignant melanoma by 11 times.

How does sunlight cause melanoma?

What is it about sunlight that might cause such a lethal change in the skin? The fault lies not in the sunshine we can see, but the 'hidden' ultraviolet that our eyes don't register. It stimulates the cells in the basal layer of the skin to produce chemicals called growth factors, which reduce our immune defences and produce subtle changes in our DNA – the key chemical for healthy cell reproduction. Crucial to this change is the way in which a normal cell 'dies' at the end of its useful life.

The cells in the basal layer of the skin, at the junction of the dermis and epidermis, are in constant activity, producing ever more squamous cells and melanocytes to replace those that have run their allotted course. To keep the 'production line' perfect, they have an internal mechanism that in a factory would be called quality control. Each cell can recognize when something is going wrong within it – it might be an infection or a change towards the beginning of cancer. Once it receives that 'signal', it 'commits suicide', a process called apoptosis – as we mentioned earlier. Apoptosis is also the reason that skin retains its normal shape. Cells recognize their boundaries with other tissues, and 'messenger' chemicals within them and around them make sure that they do not stray into the 'territories' of neighbouring cells. This is the rule for all organs, including the skin: apoptosis is the crucial mechanism for keeping their architecture, shape and size as they should be.

One of the actions of sunlight on the skin is to suppress apoptosis. Cells damaged by ultraviolet light can no longer recognize the early changes towards cancer, and do not obey the quality control order to die off. They therefore continue to multiply, producing more 'daughter' cells, all of which contain the same error. Before long, the normal architecture of the skin is destroyed as the non-apoptotic cells multiply faster than the cells around them, invading their space and creating a mass that stands out from the rest of the tissues. The first sign of that is a lump, or nodule, or a thickened or ulcerated area of skin that doesn't heal.

Why have we a system in the body, after millions of years of evolution, that is so vulnerable to cancerous change? To answer that, we need to understand the normal reaction of skin to sunlight. Sun on our skin 'switches on' our melanocytes to produce melanin, which acts as an internal sunscreen and protects against damage. It also switches on the basal cells to produce the squamous cells that form the outer layers of our skin, eventually becoming the keratin layer that also protects us against sun-induced damage.

So far, so good. The melanin production is controlled by a substance called melanocortin-1, or MC1R. The sun causes MC1R to stimulate the melanocytes to produce melanin. If you have inherited a particular variant in MC1R you will produce 'pheomelanin' instead of melanin. Pheomelanin does not protect the underlying skin against the sun. Instead it produces very fair skin and red hair. This is one reason for the increase in risk of melanoma in red-haired people.

The pheomelanin story is only one of many variants in skin chemistry that put some people at more risk than others of developing a melanoma. Researchers have identified other mutations, in gene systems called NRAS and BRAF, which are found in some 10–30 per cent of melanomas (depending on the researchers), which promote unrestrained growth of cells.

One benefit of this knowledge is that we are also learning about the mechanisms within the cells that protect against these changes, preventing benign naevi, for example, from turning into malignant melanomas. You will hear more in the near future about proteins formed by normal genes, called p16 and p14ARF, which may act as 'brakes' on unrestrained cell growth.

If you have relatives with melanoma, your risk of developing one is higher than normal. Apart from CDKN2A mentioned above, we know of another gene, CDK4, mutations in which stop apoptosis and promote melanoma. A site ('locus') on chromosome 1 is being studied, too, as a mutation in it has been linked with cases of melanoma – but so far the gene responsible has not been identified. Many, but not all, people with these genetic mutations have multiple 'atypical' naevi (more than 100 brown 'moles' of different sizes) on their bodies. Such numbers of moles are a pointer to susceptibility to melanoma, regardless of whether or not there is a CDKN2A mutation. The main message for you, if you have a lot of pigmented naevi, is to avoid direct contact between your skin and the sun.

The news that we now know that possession of certain gene types may make you much more susceptible than normal to malignant melanoma should not send you rushing for genetic screening. The work of the Melanoma Genetics Consortium, the body co-ordinating genetics research into families with melanoma, should still be confined to research, rather than clinical studies (Kefford and colleagues, 2002). There are three good reasons for this: the first is that even if you have a positive test for one of these melanoma-inducing genes, it is very difficult to predict whether it will become activated – there is a very low chance that you will develop a malignant melanoma; the second reason is that we still have not identified many of the genes that may cause malignancy in susceptible families, so that a negative test does not mean that you will *not* have a melanoma; the third, and probably the best, reason is that even if you are identified as a 'carrier' of the melanoma gene, we don't know what to do – apart from the usual warnings against sunburn – to minimize your chances of one developing. This message will surely change in the future as we learn more about the genetic flaws that lead to melanoma and how to block them.

In the meantime, doctors identify individuals at high risk of developing a melanoma from the list of characteristics in Table 1. They divide patients into high-, intermediate- and low-risk categories. Those at high risk (with two or more of the factors in Table 1) are educated about sun protection, regular self-examination for changes in moles and the appearance of new skin 'spots', and in very high-risk cases, regular examinations by a dermatologist. The rest of us (the vast majority) also need to know how to spot an early melanoma.

Spotting the early melanoma – yourself

The earlier you identify in your skin a potential melanoma, the greater your likelihood is of catching it before it has spread, and of a lasting cure. Today's doctors are trained to identify melanomas simply by using good lighting and a magnifying glass. You can do the same.

A 'spot' is more likely to be a melanoma if it is asymmetrical (most benign 'moles' are roughly symmetrical), has an irregular outline (see Figure 5), with a border that seems to merge imperceptibly or gradually into the surrounding skin, with variations in shades of brown, black or blue, and a diameter of more than 6 millimetres. This is the basis of the 'ABCDE' identification system for melanoma that has been used to alert people all over the world to the possibility that they may have a melanoma:

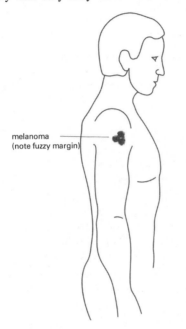

melanoma
(note fuzzy margin)

Figure 5 Melanoma

- A for asymmetry
- B for blurred outline
- C for colour variation
- D for diameter over 6 millimetres
- E for elevation above the skin surface or for enlargement from its previous size

This sounds straightforward enough, but it isn't as accurate or dependable as it appears. Let's return to Drs Strayer and Reynolds and their difficulties with this system. In their large series of patients, some lesions that would fit with many of the above criteria for malignant melanoma turned out to be one of the following (see Chapter 4 for further explanation):

- Seborrhoeic keratoses
- Injured or irritated naevi (moles)
- Pigmented basal cell cancers
- Lentigo maligna
- Blue naevi
- Angiokeratoma (a warty lesion containing blood vessels)
- Bruising
- Venous lake haemangioma (in which there are abnormally wide veins)
- Dermatofibromas
- Pigmented solar keratoses

Also, the ABCDE system doesn't pick up 'nodular' melanomas, which may be a symmetrical shape and have a well-defined smooth edge that isn't irregular, and so can be at an advanced stage before the person sees the doctor for the first time. Nodular and small melanomas may not be varied in colour, and small malignant melanomas may well metastasize before they reach 6 millimetres in diameter. So criteria ABC and D may all be absent in early melanomas. The ABCDE system also fails to take into account any recent change in appearance, which is a serious flaw.

New booklets by both the American Cancer Society and by Cancer Research UK (CRUK) have therefore abandoned the ABCDE system and replaced it with a new seven-point test. This has three major points:

- Change in size
- Change in shape
- Change in colour

And three minor signs:

- Inflammation, crusting or bleeding

- A sensory change (it feels different, and there may be pain or itching)
- A diameter of or above 7 millimetres

If you have one or more of the 'majors' and any of the 'minors', the lesion is a melanoma until proven otherwise, regardless of its size, colour or shape.

The booklets go further than simply describing the seven points. They emphasize that changes in size, shape or colour are the most important early signs of a melanoma, but add that the changes progress over a month or more, and even a year or two. Extra warning signs include new 'spots' and 'sores' that do not heal. These criteria will 'catch' small melanomas, nodular melanomas and 'amelanotic' melanomas (melanomas that are the same colour as the surrounding flesh). Nodular melanomas – the ones that remain as small round 'domes' – may well not be pigmented at all. About half of them remain pink, and this can falsely reassure people who have them that they can't be malignant. However, the seven-point system will pick them up because they have gradually grown bigger, they probably itch or may be red and 'angry', or they bleed or just feel 'different'. Melanomas that spread over the surface of the skin, in contrast, are almost always dark brown or black, and are quicker to raise their owner's concern.

The seven-point system is still not ideal on its own. Its approach to early melanoma detection is limited by the fact that people are not familiar with the size and shape of the spots on their skin, even when they were born with them. That old saying, 'I know it like the back of my hand', is quite inaccurate. Shut your eyes now and imagine the back of your hand, in detail. Think of where the veins are, how long your fingers are, where any sun-related spots or freckles are and their size. Then open your eyes. You will be surprised how inaccurate you were. Now shut your eyes again and think of all the spots you have on your body and limbs. Then look at yourself in a full-length mirror. Apart from your face, with which you are very familiar, how accurate were you on the appearance of moles, freckles and other blemishes on your skin? Remember you were interested enough to have bought or borrowed this book, yet you are probably wildly out on the appearance of your skin. Now think of people who are less interested – how accurate will they be?

So accepting that you have less than optimum awareness of the state of your skin, what should you do about it? Here is Dr Weinstock again. He wrote in 1999 and in 2004 that between 10 and 20 per cent only of the population of the USA thoroughly inspect their skin each month to check on any change in their 'spots' or on any new lesions (Weinstock, 2004). He stresses that it is of little use to exhort people to look out for changes in their skin without also teaching them to examine it thoroughly and regularly. So far, the message does not seem to have been heeded: Dr Weinstock reported no substantial improvement in skin health awareness in the USA, despite the many public health messages in the media and from doctors. As Dr Weinstock says, the early detection of melanoma ultimately relies on the combined efforts of specialists, generalists and the public.

Spotting the early melanoma – how the doctor does it

When the doctor is in doubt about whether or not the lesion is a melanoma, the most accurate way is to arrange an 'excision biopsy'. The whole lesion is removed, with a definite margin of normal skin all around it, and the specimen examined under a microscope.

Before that, however, the doctor may use 'skin surface imaging' to examine it in detail. The instrument both magnifies the lesion and applies either polarized light or uses a film of liquid that prevents scattering of light at the skin surface. This 'epiluminescence' makes it possible to see the smallest detail of the lesion, most of which is invisible to the naked eye.

Skin surface microscopy reveals the details of the changes in colour (there is often a blue-white 'veil' across the surface of a malignant lesion) and properties such as 'radial streaming' (in which there are streaks of melanin spreading out from the centre) and peripheral black dots (small spots of melanin outside the margin of the lesion). There are even computerized systems that examine photographs of lesions and compare their characteristics with a 'bank' of similar malignant and non-malignant lesions. The computer then judges the malignancy (or not) of the lesion under study: it is rarely wrong.

The final diagnosis – from the pathologist

The next stage, if melanoma is one of the possible diagnoses on clinical examination, is to remove the lesion. In this 'initial' surgery, the whole lesion must be removed, along with a margin around it of 2 millimetres, and the removal has to be deep enough to ensure that no underlying possibly malignant tissue is left behind. This preliminary surgery has to be as limited as possible, so that the later surgery can be planned properly, on the basis of the microscopic results. Taking too wide a margin in the first stage may make later surgery more complex. The pathologist will report on the site and type of melanoma (whether it is spreading or nodular), its thickness (this is called a Breslow thickness), whether there is ulceration, and the number of mitotic (reproducing) cells per square millimetre of the microscope field of view. The report will also comment on whether there is tumour invasion into the skin lymphatics or blood vessels, or into nerves. Among other more technical observations, the report is completed by measurement of the nearest distance of the margin of the material to any tumour tissue, both to the sides and underneath.

The subsequent treatment is based on the pathologist's report. Melanomas are 'staged' by their thickness within the skin from under 1 to over 4 millimetres, whether or not there is ulceration, and then whether there is spread to nearby lymph nodes, and finally distant metastases:

- Stage 0 is a non-malignant melanoma lying within the skin but not yet showing signs of becoming cancerous.
- Stage 1A is under 1 millimetre thick (in depth), and stage 1B is under 1 millimetre in diameter with ulceration, or from 1 to 2 millimetres thick without ulceration.
- Stage 2A is from 1 to 2 millimetres thick with ulceration, and 2B is from 2 to 4 millimetres thick without ulceration. Stage 2 C has a tumour more than 4 millimetres thick with ulceration.
- Stage 3A is defined as any tumour thickness with no ulcer but one to three regional lymph nodes (lymph glands that drain the site of the lesion) affected on microscopy. Stage 3B is a 3A tumour with ulceration, or any tumour thickness with one to three affected nodes enlarged enough for the spread to be seen with the naked eye ('macroscopic' nodes), or which has a 'satellite' tumour

nearby, but no distant spread. In stage 3C there are both microscopic and macroscopic nodes, or tumours with four or more nodes affected.

- Stage 4 is defined as any number of nodes and distant metastases.

These details are very important, because it gives your consultants an idea of what can be expected, and how you should be treated. Table 2 shows the five- and ten-year survival rates in 2002 for the four main stages. The figures were based on the details of 17,600 patients from 13 melanoma treatment centres worldwide. If you have melanoma, don't be shocked by these figures: they are improving all the time, especially now that new treatments are under way for stage 4 disease. They do emphasize, however, how important it is to seek your doctor's help early if you have any suspicion at all that you have skin cancer. You have a much better chance of surviving your cancer in stages 1 and 2 than in stages 3 and 4.

Table 2 Melanoma survival rates, 2002

	5-year survival (%)	10-year survival (%)
Stage 1 (tumour 1 millimetre thick or less)	93	85
Stage 2 (tumour more than 1 millimetre thick)	68	55
Stage 3 (spread to regional nodes)	45	36
Stage 4 (metastases to distant sites)	11	6

Source: American Joint Committee on Cancer (AJCC), *Staging Manual*, 6th edn, 2002.

Do remember, too, that many of the 17,600 people from whom these figures were calculated were older, and that the five- and ten-year survival figures for those in stage 1 are very similar to the figures for the normal population of the same age. We all have to die eventually, and more than 80 per cent of people with melanoma die from other causes than their cancer (Beddingfield, 2003). The survivors are mainly in stages 1 and 2, but there are many from stages 3 and 4. Virtually all stage 1 melanomas are completely cured today.

Further investigations

Given that you have been told that you have melanoma, what next step can you expect? Again it depends on your stage.

For stage 1

Happily, the vast majority of people who are told that they have malignant melanoma are in stage 1. They have a small tumour that has not spread and is only present at the spot on the skin for which they have asked their doctor's advice. There is probably no reason for them to have further tests. Naturally, if you are given a stage 1 diagnosis you will still be worried about whether there might be distant spread that the doctor can't detect simply on a normal examination, so you will be expecting further tests to remove that doubt.

However, there's no evidence that they will remove that doubt. The analyses of further test results in several large studies of cases of stage 1 melanoma strongly suggest that they only complicate things for the patients, raising unwarranted doubts rather than settling them.

For example, chest X-rays showed metastases (secondary tumours) in only 1 of 876 consecutive people with stage 1 melanoma – around 1 in 1,000 cases. In contrast, 15 per cent of the 876 were asked to return because of initial doubts about the X-rays – doubts that turned out to be groundless (Terhune and colleagues, 1998). These are termed 'false positives', and are a source of unnecessary anxiety for the patients and wasted time and expense for the hospital and staff.

Computer-assisted tomography (CAT scans) fares no better. In one large series, in only 1.3 per cent of the newly diagnosed did the scan find evidence of metastases, but there was a 15.8 per cent false positive rate (Buzaid and colleagues, 1993). Bone scans, nuclear medicine scans, liver scans and brain scans have even lower positive rates for distant spread, and positron emission tomography (PET scans) are too insensitive to detect early spread into regional nodes, so are not recommended for people thought to have stage 1 disease.

To summarize, if your doctors think you have stage 1 melanoma you will have the tumour completely removed, you will have no more tests, and you can return home secure in the feeling that you are cured.

For later stages

If your melanoma is more than 4 millimetres in depth, then you may be asked to have a CAT scan before you are asked to undergo the next stage of surgery. This second surgical stage involves removing a wider rim of the skin around where the tumour has been removed, and clearance of the regional lymph nodes (to try to ensure complete removal of all melanoma tissue in stage 2 patients). The CAT scan is needed to rule out any distant metastases, as they would make the second operation inappropriate, and you would then proceed to medical treatments.

If you do have metastases, then you will need the correct scans to identify where they are and their size. The choice includes CAT, MRI (magnetic resonance imaging) and PET (positron emission tomography). Much depends on the hospital's preference and on the specialist team's experience, as well as on the extent and location of your metastases. It is important to know where the metastases are, because the oncology team need to be able to compare the initial findings with the results after treatment. It is also a boost for you to know that your tumours are shrinking, and that you still have much to look forward to.

The next step in your care is to decide on treatment. That depends on the stage of your disease: the various strategies are described in Chapter 9.

9

Treating malignant melanoma – today's choices

So you have had your melanoma removed in the initial surgery for staging and, along with most other people with melanoma, you have been told that your lesion was in stage 1. What happens next? You now have to undergo a second operation, this time taking away a rim of skin 2 centimetres wide. It has taken many years, and studies of thousands of people with melanoma in trials conducted by the World Health Organization Melanoma Program, the Swedish Melanoma Study, the French Group for Research on Malignant Melanoma, the United States Intergroup Melanoma Surgical Trial and the United Kingdom Melanoma Study Group Trial to come to the conclusion that 2 centimetres is a wide enough margin to remove around most melanomas in order to avoid leaving behind microscopic metastases and spread. For melanomas that are 1 millimetre or less in depth (as determined by the initial surgery), the margin needs only to be 1 centimetre, but for all other melanomas a 2-centimetre zone is needed. A balance has to be struck between the disfigurement caused by taking a wider margin and the small possibility that the narrower skin removal will leave behind a tiny amount of cancerous material.

Once you have had the second operation, and you have been given the all-clear by the pathologist and surgeon, you are considered disease-free. However, that's not the end of your story. Because you are still at risk of a relapse around the site, or of a metastasis elsewhere, you will be asked to return for follow-up. At the minimum, that means a visit once a year to the clinic to check your skin and to feel for any enlarged nodes. If you are at high risk of further melanomas because you have a multitude of moles or relatives with melanoma, you will be recalled earlier.

Sentinel node samples

You may be asked for a 'sentinel node' sample. The idea is a simple one. Lymph draining from a melanoma site first flows towards a 'sentinel' node – the first lymph node along the vessel. Nodes are areas packed with lymphocytes, white blood and tissue cells that are our first defence against infection with bacteria or viruses and against metastatic cancer cells arriving from the area of skin they serve. Think of tonsillitis when you were young. You probably had with it a painful swelling down the side of your neck under the ear. That was your sentinel node from the tonsil reacting to the infection. In the same way, your sentinel node from the melanoma fights off the arrival of the 'daughter' cancer cells.

Studies of nodes draining sites of cancers show that they are the first sites of distant spread from the tumour, and they 'hold up' the travelling tumour cells for some time before there is any distant metastasis beyond them. So if there is any spread from the primary site, the sentinel node will be the first port of call. If your sentinel node contains no tumour cells, then you can fairly safely assume that you are free of spread of melanoma. It can be a big relief to get that welcome news.

When sampling of sentinel nodes started in the early 1990s, the investigators used injections of a blue dye to find the node and then removed it to examine the cells microscopically. Today, the sentinel node team of an experienced surgeon, a nuclear medicine radiologist and a pathologist work together to identify nodes using an injection of radioactive technetium along with the dye. This is extremely accurate at defining the site of the 'sentinel'. The nuclear medicine specialist prepares the radioactive material, the surgeon removes the node, and the pathologist uses his or her skills to stain the node material in such a way that every trace of cancerous material from the tumour can be found.

Your likelihood of having a metastasis in your sentinel node is only 1 per cent if your tumour is under 0.8 millimetres thick. It is 8 per cent if it is between 0.8 and 1.5 millimetres thick, 23 per cent if it is between 1.5 and 4 millimetres thick, and 36 per cent if it is thicker than 4 millimetres (Bleicher and colleagues, 2003). As your chances of long-term survival relate closely to the presence of metastases in the sentinel node, this is a very important investigation. It is a powerful argument for reporting as early as possible any enlarging 'spot' that could possibly be a melanoma, and before it begins to thicken within your skin or raise itself above the level of the surrounding skin.

Sentinel node sampling is a small operation, with little in the way of side effects, and the wound usually heals quickly. Even so, it can cause complications with healing and discomfort in around 4 per cent of people, so it is not completely without risk. Because of this, and because of the very low rate of spread to nodes from tumours less than 1 millimetre thick, sentinel node sampling is not proposed for patients with such small melanomas. Only if the pathologist sees features in the initial melanoma that suggest it is more likely than others of similar size to metastasize early would you be offered it for a small tumour. However, most melanoma surgeons will ask you to give consent for sentinel node sampling if your primary tumour is thicker than 1 millimetre.

There are two possible outcomes to your sample. The first is a negative result, which gives you confidence that you are probably cured. If the result is positive for melanoma spread, then you will be considered for 'adjuvant' (extra) medical treatment. Although this isn't the best news, at least you can be reassured that you are getting the full treatment for your tumour, and that every effort is being made to eradicate it.

The Sydney Melanoma Unit followed up their results of people with melanoma subjected to sentinel node sampling (Ka and colleagues, 2004). The five-year survival rate of the 846 whose sentinel nodes were free of melanoma was 90 per cent, and for the 145 people with spread to their sentinel nodes it was 56 per cent. This is extremely helpful, because it meant that 846 patients did not need any further treatment, and that the team could concentrate their efforts on the 145 who did need special attention and extra management of their tumours.

Adjuvant treatment

The choice of adjuvant treatment has included in the past chemotherapy (using synthetic anti-cancer drugs), vaccines, biological drugs and combinations of them all. The only treatment to show definite benefit, in that it does change the progression of the disease, is high-dose interferon-alpha. In an analysis of several trials in the USA, giving it to sentinel node-positive patients improved the numbers who were free of relapse at five years by 10 per cent. It is the only approved adjuvant for this purpose in the USA, but the researchers are looking for even better results. Current trials are combining vaccines derived from melanoma cells given alone or with a series of cytokines, including substances called interleukin 2, granulocyte-macrophage colony-stimulating factor and interferon-alpha, and others are including cytotoxic anti-cancer drugs in the 'mix'.

All these trials have the aim of reducing the burden of melanoma cells in the body and possibly preventing distant metastases. They are unpleasant to tolerate at the time, but they may well prolong your life and give you hope for the long-term future.

Removing more nodes

If you do have obvious spread (for example, you can feel a lump in an armpit) to regional lymph nodes (the next 'stopping-off point' for the cancer after the sentinel node), then your surgeon will wish to perform a complete regional node dissection. The aim of this surgery is to clear the whole lymphatic drainage system from your melanoma of any possible metastases. This can mean surgery in the groin if the melanoma was on a leg, or in the armpit if it was on an arm, or in the neck if it was on the face. Although the surgery is not pleasant, it is worthwhile. Between 13 and 59 per cent of people undergoing regional node dissection have no further metastatic disease, and are cured (Balch and colleagues, 2001). If they had not had the surgery, the mortality rate would approach 100 per cent. Adding radiotherapy may further improve the success rate, and trials are in progress to measure the extra benefit it may offer.

Going for the distant metastases

Even if the disease has penetrated beyond the regional nodes, there can still be hope. Those with spread in up to three sites in the abdomen and chest may be offered surgery to remove them. In the past, any spread to a distant site like this was considered a death sentence, and it was thought that surgery would make no difference to the person's long-term outcome. There is plenty of evidence to abandon that viewpoint for one which allows a much more active plan of treatment. Two reports (Harpole and colleagues, 1992; Tafra and colleagues, 1994) have shown that more than 20 per cent of those who have had secondary melanomas removed from their lungs survived for a further five years. After that time, they could be considered cured. Without the surgery, their five-year survival would have been close to zero. There is even better survival after removal of secondary melanoma deposits from the bowel, with five-year survival after the surgery ranging from 28 per cent to 41 per cent (Ollila and colleagues, 1996; Krige and colleagues, 1996). Even if cure cannot be expected, sometimes removing the bulk of a mass of secondary tumours in the abdomen can greatly improve people's enjoyment of life.

Secondary melanomas in the brain or in bones are best treated with, and often respond favourably to, radiotherapy (Fife and colleagues, 2004; Stevens, 2004).

Isolating a limb

A few people with melanoma of a leg or arm develop a 'shower' of obvious metastases in the surrounding skin, but without any sign of secondary spread beyond the limb. They are suitable for 'isolated limb perfusion or infusion'. In perfusion, the circulation to and from the limb is taken over by a bypass circuit (hence 'isolation') which is then used to deliver to it, and then carry away from it, an anti-cancer drug in a high dose that would not have been tolerable were it given to the rest of the body. It is very complex surgery, but it has been reported to give complete response rates of 50 per cent or better.

Infusion is a simpler technique developed from perfusion, and has been reported to give similar results by the same surgical group (Thompson and colleagues, 1998).

Is the future immunotherapy?

Could the answer to metastatic melanoma, or indeed other primary melanomas, be immunotherapy? Melanoma has a strength that is also its weakness. Its strength is that its cells can mount a significant defence against our normal immune responses. That is why they are cancer cells – they are no longer within the control of the signals to 'commit suicide' (apoptosis), or confined to their pre-determined organ shape by neighbouring cells putting out cytokines against them. So they spread locally and distantly.

Their weakness is that we know a great deal, and are learning every day more and more, about the details of melanoma chemistry, and can visualize ways of overcoming it – in effect, turning it back into a normal cell that obeys the rules. That is the aim of immunotherapy.

Melanoma cells have three main ways of defeating our attacks on them. They have a way of making our immune systems tolerate their abnormal chemistry – a property called host tolerance. Melanoma cells also produce chemicals that suppress our immune reaction against them. And they form clones of cells (exact replicas of the original cancer cells) that have lost their ability to undergo apoptosis. All of these properties make it easier for the cells to spread both locally and distantly, and to survive much longer than normal melanocytes. They are also properties that can be targeted by new treatments.

One target is the system of 'regulatory T-cells'. These are white blood cells (lymphocytes) that have passed through the thymus gland (hence the T), during which time they become active in regulating various other cell mechanisms. One of their duties is to 'switch off' another group of white cells called T-killer cells, whose job is to detect and kill tumour cells. So the researchers are studying new drugs that will eliminate regulatory T-cell activity, allowing the T-killer cells to destroy the melanoma cells.

A second approach involves the making of 'monoclonal antibodies' (one is called MDX-010) that will switch off the immune-suppressant 'signal' put out by the melanoma cell. That will allow the immune system to do its job, and deal with the intruder. A third system is to 'expand' the person's population of tumour-specific T-killer cells, and to improve their chances of success by combining the system with aggressive chemotherapy.

Writing in 2006, I have high hopes that the immunotherapy approach will succeed, but it will take time.

Chemotherapy and biological treatment

I am less optimistic about chemotherapy, although I will be very glad to be proved wrong. It is reserved for people with advanced melanoma, and the current single-drug treatments (drug names are dacarbazine, temozolomide and fotemustine) are used mainly because they are simple to use and are relatively free of severe side effects, unlike more toxic combination treatments (using three drugs, plus interferon and interleukin), which are no more successful than the single-drug treatments. Only a minority of people respond well to them, some trials reporting response rates as low as 10 per cent.

Perhaps biological treatment will be more effective. The biological pharmaceutical company Genta Incorporated, of New Jersey, USA, has developed 'oblimersen'; this is an 'oligonucleotide', a natural constituent of a cell that attacks the specific substance Bcl-2 that melanoma cells produce in abundance. We now know that Bcl-2 is an 'anti-apoptotic' molecule. It is the substance that stops the cancer cell from 'committing suicide'. If oblimersen can succeed in knocking out Bcl-2, the melanoma cells should die off of their own accord.

Oblimersen may not be the complete answer, but it is a very good start, and we can look forward to more treatments like it. Treatments like oblimersen, and another named BAY 43-9006, which was reported upon in 2004, may have to be given along with chemotherapy for the best results, but the signs are hopeful that we are at the birth of a new form of medical treatment for widespread cancer. The future is good, not bleak, in the fight against melanoma.

10

Mycosis fungoides – Ashley Medicks's story

When I thought about writing this book, I wondered how I could encourage people with mycosis fungoides (MF). As mentioned in Chapter 1, it is the disease that killed the actor Paul Eddington. Essentially, it is a cancer of the lymphocytes in the skin, and it has so far proved to be incurable. I couldn't see a way of describing it in a form that would encourage those with MF to look forward and to have hope.

That was before I heard of Ashley Medicks. He runs Skinship UK, a self-help group for all people with skin problems, from a small cottage in Dumfriesshire. He has had MF for 35 years. His body is covered with thickened scaly patches and plaques, and he is in constant discomfort.

Ashley is a survivor. When as a young adult he was told he had the disease, he decided to learn all about it. Given a short prognosis by his dermatologist, and knowing that he probably faced an uncomfortable death, he changed his life completely. He and his wife spent two years travelling round Africa, where incidentally he was probably exposed to a lot more sunlight than he had been used to. That in itself may have helped him: ultraviolet light is a treatment, not a danger, for mycosis fungoides. He followed a Mediterranean diet, eating the right foods to give his immune system the best chance of fighting his disease. He moved from his busy London life to rural Scotland, where people naturally seem to live longer than in the city. He learned that selenium supplements might improve his skin's health, and has taken a 250-milligram tablet a day for some years. He thinks it has helped.

But the main reason I'm writing is not about Ashley's own illness, remarkable as his story is. More astounding is the way he has reacted to it. In Skinship he has become a one-man organization to help people with skin diseases, not just from MF, but also other skin cancers, and chronic skin diseases such as eczema, psoriasis and acne. He has the support of his local dermatologist and of the British Dermatology Association, and the enthusiasm of two highly respected people in the public eye, Dr Mark Porter and Ben Elton, behind him. He is a stakeholder (a non-medical adviser) for skin cancer in NICE, the UK's National Institute for Clinical Excellence, and when I last spoke to Ashley he was wading through the latest NICE guidelines on the management of melanoma – a document over 800 pages long.

As long ago as December 1994, Ashley appeared on BBC2's *Open Space* programme, which dealt with the uncomfortable relationships between those with skin conditions and the general public. He told me how difficult it was for people with MF, psoriasis or eczema to strip off in public – for example, at a swimming pool. It was mainly his efforts that made it illegal for those with skin conditions to be ejected from a pool on the basis of objections from others who are offended by their appearance and the fear that they might be 'infected' by them. Attitudes like that change slowly, and we need people like Ashley to accelerate the change.

Ashley supports the German health authorities for sending, at government expense, people with skin conditions to Dead Sea resorts for weeks at a time as part of their treatment. The atmosphere in the evenings in these resorts is electric, as people realize for the first time in their adult lives they are not being looked upon with distaste or horror. It is much cheaper to send them to Israel than to admit them to hospital, and the end-results are better – not just in improved health, but in enjoyment too.

He has also tackled the problem of itch. Ashley describes the 'itch-scratch' syndrome that makes life hell for MF and those with eczema. The urge to scratch is overwhelming, but its result is to irritate the skin even more, and for the itch to return with even greater intensity. People with itch don't realize how often they scratch. Ashley tells of Sue Armstrong Brown who, given a 'clicker' to count the number of times a day she scratched her eczematous skin, was astonished at a score of several hundreds. If people can be persuaded to stop scratching, and to use anti-irritant creams, they can break the vicious cycle, and their skin conditions will improve. Ashley recommends Sue's book, *The Eczema Solution* (published by Vermilion), in which she describes how to break the itch-scratch cycle within six weeks.

A main part of the anti-itch treatment has been to find a cream against itch that really works, will not make the problems worse, and is inexpensive. In 2005 he persuaded Boots the Chemists to market a mixture of 2 per cent menthol in aqueous cream as an anti-itching cream for chronic itch. Many dermatologists support him in doing so.

Ashley feels that having MF has made him a better person. Obviously he would have much preferred to have normal skin, but his disease made him change his priorities, and he would not abandon his present lifestyle to return to his old London-based city business life, with its constant mental and physical stresses. He lives in an idyllic country area that I know well, living as I do in a neighbouring county. It contributes to his sense of well-being, and perhaps to his much longer life than expected. He pays great tribute to the love and care of his wife, Jackie, who has supported him throughout his long years of life-threatening illness, and without whom he feels he could not have survived. He welcomes calls from anyone with skin problems, particularly from those with MF and the more common skin cancers, and is happy for me to include his phone number here (tel. 01387 760567). You will find yourself speaking to a most remarkable, cheerful, courageous and happy man.

11
Getting help

Living with cancer raises many questions, and there never seems to be enough time with your doctor to ask them all. You may even feel embarrassed at taking up their time, knowing how busy they seem to be. Yet the doctors and cancer specialists I know would be only too happy to explain things in more detail or to answer awkward questions, if you would ask them. Even a busy man or woman can always find time for you.

So if you wish to know more about your cancer, the first person to talk to is your doctor, your dermatologist, your oncologist or your cancer nurse. They are all well trained in dealing with people with cancers, and you will find them sympathetic and friendly. In today's atmosphere of openness, they will tell you the truth but they will never leave you without hope.

There are many charities to whom to turn for information and support:

CancerBACUP
3 Bath Place
Rivington Street
London EC2A 3JR
Tel.: 020 7739 2280 (general enquiries)
Helpline: 0808 800 1234 (for urgent enquiries; helpline staffed by cancer nurses, 9 am to 8 pm, Mondays to Fridays)
Website: www.cancerbacup.org.uk

Supplies information and support for people with cancer, their families and friends.

Cancerlink
89 Albert Embankment
London SE1 7UQ
Tel.: 020 7840 7840
Support line: 0808 808 2020 (9 am to 6 pm, Mondays to Fridays)
Website: www.cancerlink.org

Part of Macmillan Cancer Relief (see below): a directory of more than 700 cancer self-help and support groups.

Lymphoma Association
PO Box 386
Aylesbury
Bucks HP20 2GA
Tel.: 01296 619 400
Helpline: 0808 808 5555
Website: www.lymphoma.org.uk

Gives specialized information about all kinds of lymphoma, including mycosis fungoides. It produces a regular newsletter, videos, booklets and leaflets about lymphoma, and has associated local groups throughout the country.

Macmillan Cancer Relief
89 Albert Embankment
London SE1 7UQ
Tel.: 0808 808 2020 (freephone, 9 am to 6 pm, Mondays to Fridays)
Website: www.macmillan.org.uk
Email: cancerline@macmillan.org.uk

Funds specialist Macmillan nurses and doctors, buildings for cancer treatment and care, and grants for patients in financial difficulties.

MARC'S Line (Melanoma And Related Cancers of the Skin)
Tel.: 01722 415071 (9 am to 5 pm, Mondays to Fridays)
Website: www.wessexcancer.org/marcsline

Part of Wessex Cancer Trust and affiliated to the Dermatology Treatment Centre at Salisbury District Hospital in Wiltshire. Helpline and resource centre, involved in education about skin cancer through providing leaflets and factsheets.

Marie Curie Cancer Care
89 Albert Embankment
London SE1 7UQ
Tel.: 020 7599 7777
Website: www.mariecurie.org.uk

Provides care in patients' homes and in 11 centres throughout the UK. Also strongly supports cancer research.

Skinship
C/o Ashley Medicks
Plascow Cottage
Kirkgunzeon
Dumfries DG2 8JT
Tel.: 01387 760567
Website: www.ukselfhelp.info/skinship

He is pleased to help anyone in trouble, and is always up to date with his information, which is fully in line with modern treatments for cancers. This includes the 800-plus pages outlining the NICE guidelines.

References

American Journal of Preventive Medicine, vol. 38, June 2004, pp. 761–5.

Balch, C. M. and colleagues, *Journal of Clinical Oncology*, vol. 19, 2001, pp. 3622–34.

Beddingfield, F. C., *Oncologist*, vol. 8, 2003, pp. 459–65.

Berwick, M. and colleagues, *Journal of the National Cancer Institute*, vol. 97[3], 2 February 2005, pp. 195–99.

Bigby, M. E., in *Archives of Dermatology* (American Medical Association publication), June 2004.

Bleicher, R. J. and colleagues, *Journal of Clinical Oncology*, vol. 21, 2003, pp. 1326–31.

Buzaid, A. C. and colleagues, *Journal of Clinical Oncology*, vol. 11, 1993, pp. 638–43.

Cantorna, M. T. and Mahon, B. D., *Experimental Biological Medicine*, vol. 229(11), December 2004, pp. 1136–42.

Cornell, R. C. and colleagues, *Journal of the American Academy of Dermatology*, vol. 23, 1990, pp. 694–700.

De Sevaux, R. G. and colleagues, *Journal of the American Academy of Dermatology*, vol. 49, 2003, pp. 407–12.

Fife, K. M. and colleagues, *Journal of Clinical Oncology*, vol. 22, 2004, pp. 1293–1300.

Giovannucci, E., in *Cancer Causes*, vol. 167(2), March 2005, pp. 83–95.

Grant, W. B., writing in *Cancer*, vol. 94(6), 15 March 2002, pp. 1867–75.

Greenway, H. T. and colleagues, *Journal of the American Academy of Dermatology*, vol. 15, 1986, pp. 437–43.

Hall, V. L. and colleagues, *Clinical Radiology*, vol. 37, 1986, pp. 33–4.

Harpole, D. H. and colleagues, *Journal of Thoracic and Cardiovascular Surgery*, vol. 103, 1992, pp. 743–8.

Harwood, C. A. and colleagues, *Journal of Clinical Pathology*, vol. 52, 1999, pp. 249–53.

Heston, J. F. and colleagues, vol. 70, National Cancer Institute

Monographs 1986, p. 347.

Holman, C. D. J. and Armstrong, B. K., *Journal of the National Cancer Institute*, vol. 73, 1984, pp. 75–82.

Ka, V. S. K. and colleagues, *Annals of Surgical Oncology*, vol. 11, 2004, p. S60.

Kefford, R. and colleagues, *Lancet Oncology*, vol. 3, 2002, pp. 653–4.

Khlat, M. and colleagues, *American Journal of Epidemiology*, vol. 135, 1992, pp. 1103–13.

Krige, J. E. and colleagues, *American Surgery*, vol. 62, 1996, pp. 658–63.

Mohs, F. E., *Archives of Surgery*, vol. 42, 1941, pp. 279–95.

Mohs, F. E., *Archives of Dermatology*, vol. 112, 1976, pp. 211–15.

Motley, R., Kersey, P. and Lawrence, C., *British Journal of Plastic Surgery*, vol. 56, 2003, pp. 85–91.

Ollila, D. W. and colleagues, *Archives of Surgery*, vol. 131, 1996, pp. 975–80.

Peris, K. and colleagues, *New England Journal of Medicine*, vol. 341, 1999, pp. 1767–8.

Polednak, A. P., Cancer Incidence in Connecticut: Connecticut Tumour Registry, 2001.

Rowe, D. E. and colleagues, *Journal of Dermatological and Surgical Oncology*, vol. 15, 1989, pp. 315–18 and pp. 424–31.

Shearman, J. C., *British Medical Journal*, vol. 1, 1978, p. 283.

Stevens, G. N., *Textbook of Melanoma*, London, Martin Dunitz, pp. 395–403.

Strayer, S. M., report on the diagnosis of skin cancers, *Journal of Family Practice*, University of Virginia Health Service, in Charlottesville, vol. 52, March 2003.

Swerdlow, A. J. and colleagues, *British Journal of Cancer*, vol. 72, 1995, pp. 236–43.

Tafra, L. and colleagues, *Journal of Thoracic and Cardiovascular Surgery*, vol. 110, 1994, pp. 119–28.

Terhune, M. H. and colleagues, *Archives of Dermatology*, vol. 134, 1998, pp. 569–72.

Thieden, L. and colleagues, *Journal of Investigative Dermatology*, vol. 123, 2004, pp. 1147–50.

Thompson, J. F. and colleagues, *Seminars in Surgical Oncology*, vol. 14, 1998, pp. 238–47.

REFERENCES

Thompson, J. F. and colleagues, of the University of Sydney melanoma unit, writing in the *Lancet*, vol. 365, 19 February 2005, pp. 687–701.

Weinstock, M., *The Journal of Investigative Dermatology*, vol. 123(6), 2004, pp. 17–19.

Index